Practical Psychology for Diabetes Clinicians

How to Deal With the Key Behavioral Issues Faced by Patients and Health-Care Teams

EDITORS
Barbara J. Anderson, PhD
Richard R. Rubin, PhD, CDE

EDITORIAL ASSISTANT
Laura E. Crescenzi

REVIEWERS
Gary R. Geffken, PhD
Wylie L. McNabb, EdD
Elizabeth Walker, RN, CDE
Tim Wysocki, PhD

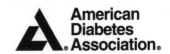
American
Diabetes
Association.

CHIEF SCIENTIFIC AND MEDICAL OFFICER
Richard Kahn, PhD

PUBLISHER
Susan H. Lau

EDITORIAL DIRECTOR
Peter Banks

ACQUISITIONS EDITOR
Susan Reynolds

BOOK EDITOR
Karen Lombardi Ingle

PRODUCTION DIRECTOR
Carolyn R. Segree

Library of Congress Cataloging-in-Publication Data

Practical psychology for diabetes clinicians : how to deal with the
  key behavioral issues faced by patients and health-care teams /
  editors, Barbara J. Anderson, Richard R. Rubin.
     p.   cm. — (Practical approaches in diabetes care)
  Includes bibliographical references and index.
   ISBN 0-945448-73-2
   1. Diabetes—Psychological aspects.   2. Clinical health
psychology.   I. Anderson, Barbara J. (Barbara Jane), 1947–
II. Rubin, Richard R.   III. American Diabetes Association.
IV. Series
     [DNLM: 1. Diabetes Mellitus—psychology.   2. Diabetes Mellitus—
therapy.   WK 810 P895 1996]
RC660.P725   1996
616.4'62'0019—dc20
DNLM/DLC
for Library of Congress   96-15937
                                                                              CIP

American Diabetes Association, Inc,
1660 Duke Street, Alexandria, VA 22314

TABLE OF CONTENTS

FOREWORD   **vii**

I *Developmental and Family Factors*

1. Working With Diabetic Children   **3**
    Alan M. Delamater, PhD

2. Working With Diabetic Adolescents   **13**
    Richard R. Rubin, PhD, CDE

3. Improving Diabetes Control in Adolescents
    With Type I Diabetes   **23**
    Joseph I. Wolfsdorf, MB, BCh

4. Caring for Elderly Patients With Diabetes   **35**
    John F. Zrebiec, MSW

5. Involving Family Members in Diabetes
    Treatment   **43**
    Barbara J. Anderson, PhD

II *Treatment Regimen Factors*

6. Dealing With Diabetes Self-Management   **53**
    *Russell E. Glasgow, PhD, and Elizabeth G.
    Eakin, PhD*

7. Eating and Diabetes: A Patient-Centered
   Approach   63
   David G. Schlundt, PhD, James W. Pichert, PhD,
   Becky Gregory, RD, and Dianne Davis, RD

8. Motivating Patients With Diabetes to Exercise   73
   David G. Marrero, PhD, and Jill M. Sizemore,
   MS

9. Helping Patients Understand and Recognize
   Hypoglycemia   83
   Linda Gonder-Frederick, PhD, Daniel J. Cox,
   PhD, and William L. Clarke, MD

10. Helping Patients Reduce Severe Hypoglycemia   93
    Daniel J. Cox, PhD, Linda Gonder-Frederick,
    PhD, and William L. Clarke, MD

III

Complex and Chronic Behavioral Issues

11. Improving Glycemic Control in Patients
    With Type I Diabetes   105
    Alan M. Jacobson, MD

12. Improving Weight Loss and Maintenance in
    Patients With Diabetes   113
    Rena R. Wing, PhD

13. Smoking Cessation in Diabetes   121
    Edwin B. Fisher, Jr, PhD, Sheryl L. Ziff, MA, and
    Debra Haire-Joshu, PhD, RN

14. Preventing Eating Disorders in Young Women
    With Type I Diabetes   133
    Wendy Satin Rapaport, PsyD, Annette M.
    LaGreca, PhD, and Paula Levine, PhD

15. Recognizing and Managing Depression in
    Patients With Diabetes   143
    Patrick J. Lustman, PhD, Linda S. Griffith, MSW,
    and Ray E. Clouse, MD

IV Prevention of Special Problems

16. Emotional Responses to Diagnosis   **155**
    Richard R. Rubin, PhD, CDE, and
    Mark Peyrot, PhD

17. Using the Empowerment Approach to Help Patients
    Change Behavior   **163**
    Robert M. Anderson, EdD, Martha M. Funnell,
    MS, RN, CDE, and Marilynn S. Arnold, MS,
    RD, CDE

18. Understanding and Treating Provider Burnout   **173**
    Cindy L. Hanson, PhD

19. Understanding and Treating Patients With
    Diabetes Burnout   **183**
    William H. Polonsky, PhD, CDE

AFTERWORD   **193**

INDEX   **195**

FOREWORD

Over the past decade, clinicians have seen the development of revolutionary technologies and treatments for diabetes. There has also been a striking—though much less visible—growth in information about the behavioral side of diabetes. This book, developed by The Council on Behavioral Medicine and Psychology of the American Diabetes Association, provides practical clinical applications of the latest behavioral information on diabetes management. We asked leading behavioral science researchers in diabetes to translate their findings into guidelines for physicians, nurses, dietitians, mental health professionals, and exercise physiologists who care for people with diabetes.

We divided this book into four areas of clinically important behavioral issues. These four areas are 1) recommendations specific to developmental (age-related) and family factors; 2) guidelines concerning treatment regimen factors; 3) recommendations for handling complex and chronic behavioral issues; and 4) guidelines for preventing special problems with the patient-physician relationship, emotional responses to diagnosis, "patient burnout," and "provider burnout."

Within each of these four areas are guidelines for handling some of the most stubborn and serious problems facing diabetes clinicians and their patients—problems such as hypoglycemia, lack of motivation, lack of exercise, excess weight, and smoking.

Psychology has a profound and permanent impact to make on the diabetes community. We hope this book serves as a useful tool for diabetes clinicians by making the latest psychological knowledge attainable and applicable.

Barbara J. Anderson, PhD
Richard R. Rubin, PhD, CDE

DEVELOPMENTAL AND FAMILY FACTORS | I

C hapters in this first section present issues facing the clinician who cares for diabetes patients in any of the three most challenging age-groups—children, adolescents, and the elderly.

In the first chapter of this section, Delamater provides practical recommendations concerning the care of pediatric patients, who are, in many ways, the most vulnerable of people with diabetes. The idea that parents are the appropriate patient when diabetes occurs in a child is addressed, and key problems in the family management of childhood diabetes are discussed.

Next, Rubin presents guidelines for working with adolescents and dealing with adolescent behavior and feelings. Strategies to maintain partnerships between adolescents and care providers as well as between adolescents and their parents are provided.

Wolfsdorf discusses the key factors involved in improving metabolic control during this most difficult developmental period. Strategies for improving glycemic control during the complex adolescent years take on extra importance when coupled with findings from the Diabetes Control and Complications Trial (DCCT) that improved glycemic control can prevent or delay the long-term complications of type I diabetes.

Zrebiec discusses the many complicated physical and psychological problems facing elderly patients with diabetes, and he offers practical guidelines for giving optimal and sensitive care to these patients.

In the last chapter of this section, B. Anderson gives four practical guidelines for working with families—whether the patient is a child, an adult, or a senior citizen. Specific recommendations allow the clinician to help families work in ways that help the patient adhere to the diabetes treatment regimen.

Working With Diabetic Children | I

Alan M. Delamater, PhD

INTRODUCTION

Successful management of diabetes is always challenging, especially when working with children. Epidemiological studies indicate that the incidence of type I diabetes has increased in recent years, particularly among young children. This chapter presents treatment guidelines and principles of intervention.

TREATMENT GUIDELINES

Help Children and Parents Manage Critical Issues at Diagnosis

The diagnosis of type I diabetes represents a crisis for both children and parents. Both must

- Accept the diagnosis and its implications in a realistic way.
- Manage their own psychological response to the diagnosis.
- Learn a new set of complex skills relating to diabetes management.
- Not allow diabetes to interfere with the attainment of normal developmental tasks.

Studies have shown that in the initial period of adaptation after diagnosis, a significant number of parents (particularly mothers) become depressed and anxious. In most cases, these reactions subside within the first year. Besides having to acquire a lot of new knowledge about diabetes and its management, parents and children must master new skills and figure out how to integrate diabetes management into daily life.

Help Parents Have Realistic Expectations Concerning Their Children's Responsibility for Self-Management

Parents of very young children assume all responsibilities for diabetes management. Over time, however, children can begin to assume some responsibilities for certain aspects of self-care.

Learning to identify who is responsible for what tasks at what times is an important issue for families, because studies have shown that disagreements about these responsibilities are related to poor glycemic control.

Some research has found that parents and clinicians disagree in their estimates of the age at which children are ready for self-care independence. Findings indicate that certain self-management behaviors (insulin adjustment, in particular) depend on cognitive maturity, rather than age. Glycemic control problems are more likely when children are given self-care responsibilities that they are not yet able to handle competently.

Help Parents Facilitate Good Self-Care Attitudes and Behaviors in Their Children

Several studies of older children and adolescents have demonstrated that poor communication skills and family conflict are associated with problems of regimen adherence and glycemic control. Parents and their children must strive for effective communication to avoid and resolve conflicts. In addition, parents and children must develop a good relationship with their health-care team. A good relationship, based on trust and support, will foster agreement and understanding about exactly what the parents and children are supposed to do to manage diabetes effectively.

Help Parents and Children Learn to Avoid and to Treat Hypoglycemia

Studies have shown that children who are diagnosed before age 5 and who have more episodes of serious hypoglycemia may be at increased risk for later neurocognitive deficits. Such children should receive psycho-educational evaluations for early identification of learning problems. Because of this potential complication and the fact that young children cannot verbalize their subjective experience of hypoglycemia, parents may feel highly stressed about hypoglycemia. Thus, parents need to monitor their child's blood glucose frequently to assure themselves that their child is not hypoglycemic. Common psychological reactions of parents and children to frequent blood glucose monitoring may include feelings of anger for the child, guilt for the parent, and distress for both.

Help Parents and Children Develop Realistic Attitudes Toward Glycemic Control

Parents may get in the habit of giving evaluative messages to their children regarding the results of blood glucose monitoring. Hyperglycemia and hypoglycemia may be seen as "bad" readings. When viewed in this way, such readings are less likely to be used as feedback to solve problems and try new strategies.

Help patients use the information they collect on a daily basis to gain a better understanding of blood glucose variations; to make appropriate changes in insulin dose, diet, and activity; and to solve problems relating to glycemic control.

Parents and children may be anxious about insulin injections and dose adjustments. After an injection, many children may not want to eat within an appropriate time, causing parents to be concerned about hypoglycemia. Many young children are finicky eaters, making meal planning very challenging. Counsel parents to tell children ahead of time when meals will be served. This can be done while administering insulin. Encourage parents to then reinforce their children for eating at the appropriate time.

Children's activity levels also may vary considerably, raising the risk of either hypoglycemia or hyperglycemia, depending on baseline blood glucose, food consumed, and available insulin. Because young children have frequent viral illnesses, parents need to know how to manage the effects of such illnesses on glycemic control.

Attaining and maintaining good glycemic control are of paramount importance, especially since the Diabetes Control and Complications Trial (DCCT) has established that "tight control" is associated with reduced health risks. However, during childhood, good control is often elusive. After repeated "trials," in which blood glucose levels seem unrelated to adherence to the prescribed regimen, parents and children may begin to feel that their self-care efforts are unrelated to glycemic outcomes. Eventually, these experiences may lead to a feeling of "learned helplessness," which has been associated with poor glycemic control in youths. Because learned helplessness may lead to depression and a feeling of "why bother to try?," it is important for children to talk about their experiences with their parents and the health-care team, who can help them cope with their difficulties in adaptive ways.

Help Parents Keep Tabs on Social Adjustment and Self-Esteem in Their Children

Self-esteem and social adjustment are significant psychosocial concerns related to daily diabetes management. Parents are often quite concerned with how their child will be accepted by peers. Older children are commonly concerned about being seen as different from other children because of what their diabetes regimen requires.

WHEN TO INTERVENE

Parents and children have much to deal with at diagnosis. Although this is the time during which most diabetes education takes place, it is important to remember that anxiety interferes with learning. Everything that is taught may not be remembered. Think of education as a process that occurs over time. Experience helps to consolidate the concepts of diabetes care. Furthermore, remember that education does not necessarily lead to competencies with regimen-related skills, and that having skills does not automatically lead to behavior change.

Educate patients, teach them self-management skills, and help them succeed at changing their behavior.

At the time of diagnosis and during the first few weeks of adjustment, the child and family typically need a lot of psychological support. It is not unreasonable to consider this a crisis, requiring a crisis-intervention approach. Reassure the family that their child can go on to live a normal life, that they will be able to learn to manage diabetes effectively, and that there is a team of health-care professionals committed to helping them succeed.

After learning the most basic survival skills, the family is essentially on their own, with follow-up typically conducted at 2- to 3-month intervals, and later at 3- to 4-month intervals. Because of the honeymoon phenomenon, fairly good glycemic control can be expected during the first 2 years or so after diagnosis. When residual beta-cell activity dissipates, glycemic control may be more difficult to attain, however, and require additional education and counseling.

Rather than waiting for problems to develop, preventive approaches may be used before risk for glycemic control problems increases. Two critical times for intervention are 1) the period just after diagnosis and 2) the period just before puberty.

HOW TO INTERVENE

There is evidence for the efficacy of behavioral interventions at the two critical times noted above. In one study, families who participated in self-management training during the first 4 months after diagnosis had children with significantly better glycemic control up to 2 years after diagnosis than patients who received conventional outpatient care without self-management training.

Self-management training focused on increasing utilization of blood glucose monitoring for making behavioral changes to improve glycemic control. Specific home tests were prescribed to help patients and their families understand how food, exercise, and insulin affect blood glucose. The goal was to build family support for regimen adherence and to develop diabetes self-care strategies based on blood glucose measurements. The lessons from this study are as follows:

- Provide education and behavioral interventions over a period of several months after diagnosis, before bad habits develop.
- Provide specific exercises so that families can experience for themselves how blood glucose is affected by various factors.
- Counsel parents to use positive reinforcement to encourage appropriate regimen behaviors in their children.

In another study, a developmentally appropriate intervention was used, involving the peer group, practical applications of blood glucose monitoring, and parental counseling to establish reasonable self-care responsibilities and parental involvement. The intervention was administered at the clinic in group format, with separate groups for children and parents. Children who received this intervention had better glycemic control over an 18-month period than those treated conventionally.

Much can be applied from the extensive literature on psychological interventions for children's behavioral disorders and regimen noncompliance. Many controlled studies have demonstrated the effectiveness of parent training in effective child behavior management strategies to reduce noncompliant behaviors in children. In general, parents tend to ignore positive behaviors and attend to and inadvertently reinforce negative behaviors. Essentially, brief interventions (6 to 8 sessions) focus on teaching parents to differentially reinforce their children's behavior: positive compliant behavior is positively reinforced; minor negative behavior is ignored (extinguished); and more serious noncompliant behavior is punished (using the "time-out" technique or loss of privileges). In addition, instructions in giving commands or making requests are provided, because noncompliance in children is often associated with ineffective methods of command-giving in parents. Token economies and behavioral contracts may be used successfully to improve regimen adherence. In a token economy, specific target behaviors are rewarded with points or tokens that can be exchanged later for desired reinforcers. Behavioral contracts specify the child's responsibilities and the privileges earned contingent upon completion of tasks.

It is very important that parents of children with diabetes be instructed in effective behavior management techniques: give clear expectations, apply positive reinforcement for successful performance with the regimen, and administer consistent consequences for nonadherence. These approaches have been used successfully in a number of controlled studies of youths with diabetes. In particular, interventions using goal setting, memos, self-monitoring or charting, behavioral contracts, and social problem-solving with behavioral rehearsal have been effective in improving adherence to various components of the regimen, and sometimes in improving glycemic control as well. It is important to help older children understand which social situations are associated with adherence problems, identify appropriate strategies for prevention of these problems, and rehearse with them how to implement those strategies. Successful interventions have been conducted with individual families and also with groups of children and parents.

CONCLUSION

Successful management of diabetes in young children presents significant challenges for all involved—parents, children, and the health-care team. While optimal glycemic control is desired, it is critical that reasonable goals be established, with consideration given to the changing regimen requirements related to the process of development in the growing child. Success should be measured not only by glycemic outcomes, but also by attainment of age-appropriate regimen-related skills and responsibilities, as well as emotional, social, and academic development. Because diabetes management in children occurs within a family context, attention must be given to family functioning. Many studies have shown its importance in relationship to health behaviors and metabolic outcomes. Encourage parents to find ways to be supportive of their child's self-care efforts, while minimizing the use of nonsupportive strategies like criticizing, nagging, and arguing.

Early interventions may prevent later problems with regimen adherence and metabolic control. The months after diagnosis are an optimal time to lay the groundwork for successful self-management. Counsel parents about the importance of positive reinforcement for performance of appropriate regimen-related behaviors. Involvement of children in performing self-care behaviors can begin in early childhood, but responsibilities for these tasks must be developmentally appropriate. Treatment should include the cultivation of adaptive thinking about and coping with less than optimal glycemic outcomes, because feelings of helplessness may impact adversely on later performance of health behaviors.

Be responsive to the needs of the family, particularly in the period after diagnosis, but also throughout the course of the child's development when the needs of the child and family may not be consistent with the prescriptions offered by the team. It is essential for normal development to proceed unhindered by the demands of diabetes management. When the two become intertwined, problems will arise.

Pay attention to family conflict, poor communication between parents and children, isolation of the family from social supports, high levels of parental stress, and difficulties with children's school performance and psychosocial adjustment. Clearly, these problems and difficulties with regimen adherence and glycemic control may indicate the need for referral to a mental health professional who is knowledgeable about diabetes and its management in children.

Many of the guidelines offered here for behavioral interventions are simple, but not easy. Behavioral changes are often gradual rather than sudden and dramatic. Patience and encouragement are essential, along with reasonable expectations for success and demonstrations by the health-care team of interest and commitment to the patient and family. The principles of reinforcement are thus as applicable and important from the health-care team to the family as from the parents to the child.

BIBLIOGRAPHY

Anderson BJ, Wolf RM, Burkhart MT, Cornell RG, Bacon GE: Effects of peer-group intervention on metabolic control of adolescents with IDDM: randomized outpatient study. *Diabetes Care* 12:179–183, 1989

Barkley RA: *Defiant Children: A Clinician's Manual for Parent Training.* New York, Guilford Press, 1987

Delamater AM: Compliance interventions for children with diabetes and other chronic diseases. In *Developmental Aspects of Health Compliance Behavior.* Krasnegor NA, Ed. Hillsdale, NJ, Lawrence Erlbaum, 1993, p. 335–354

Delamater AM, Bubb J, Davis SG, Smith JA, Schmidt L, White NH, Santiago JV: Randomized prospective study of self-management training with newly diagnosed diabetic children. *Diabetes Care* 13:492–498, 1990

Johnson SB: Insulin-dependent diabetes mellitus in childhood. In *Handbook of Pediatric Psychology (second edition)*. Roberts M, Ed. New York, Guilford Press, 1995, p. 263–285

Marteau TM, Johnson M, Baum JD, Bloch S: Goals of treatment in diabetes: comparison of doctors and parents of children with diabetes. *J Behav Med* 10:33–48, 1987

Miller-Johnson S, Emery RE, Marvin RS, Clarke W, Lovinger R, Martin M: Parent-child relationships and the management of insulin-dependent diabetes mellitus. *J Consult Clin Psychol* 62:603–610, 1994

Wysocki T, Meinhold PA, Abrams KC, Barnard MU, Clarke WL, Bellando BJ, Bourgeois MJ: Parental and professional estimates of self-care independence of children and adolescents with IDDM. *Diabetes Care* 15:43–52, 1992

Working With Diabetic Adolescents | 2

Richard R. Rubin, PhD, CDE

C INTRODUCTION

linicians often place increasing responsibility for diabetes management on their adolescent patients. This is appropriate only to the degree that it accurately reflects the young person's capacity to care for himself or herself. All too often, however, diabetes care responsibilities are turned over to teenagers without adequate consideration for their readiness. Moreover, the process of encouraging independence is rarely carried out in a way most likely to be successful. Many families and clinicians expect that mature problem-solving skills will appear fully developed during adolescence, and they often move too abruptly from a parent-responsible mode to an adolescent-responsible mode, instead of promoting this transition more gradually during preadolescence. The unfortunate consequences include a high proportion of teenagers who dramatically curtail or even stop caring for their diabetes, resulting in deteriorating glycemic control, plummeting self-esteem, and burgeoning family conflict. This chapter offers guidelines for diabetes clinicians working with adolescents. These guidelines are designed to facilitate the process of helping young people learn to effectively manage their diabetes.

DON'T ENCOURAGE INDEPENDENT SELF-CARE BASED ON AGE ALONE

Until about 10 years ago, independence in diabetes care was seen as a sign of maturity or responsibility. But recent research shows something quite different. Current studies show that in families where young people are in good control of their blood glucose, the young people—regardless of their age—have continuing support with diabetes management tasks from their parents. Therefore, don't focus on a young person's age alone when thinking about what the adolescent needs to be doing in terms of independent diabetes care. Strict age guidelines don't work. For one thing, there is almost always a big difference between a teenager's *physical* capacity to master a task and the *cognitive* and *emotional* maturity required to carry out the task on a continuing basis. Not recognizing this difference is the source of tremendous frustration for the clinician and for the parents of an adolescent with diabetes. Studies have found that often the self-management tasks parents turned over to their children were not taken over by the young people; tasks such as insulin dose adjustment simply went undone.

Another problem with turning over responsibility for diabetes management based solely on the young person's age is the fact that not all youth the same age have the same capacities. Temperamental and other individual differences powerfully affect the way young people adapt to diabetes, or to any other major life challenge. Moreover, age guidelines for independent self-care don't take into account external stresses or special needs, such as family problems, learning disabilities, and a wide range of other factors. Be sure to take an adolescent's individual circumstances into account, and continue to provide the diabetes management support the adolescent needs at this time, no matter how old he or she is. Regular reevaluation of the adolescent's diabetes self-care skills and the family division of diabetes responsibilities is also worthwhile. This will guide recommendations about the appropriate transfer of responsibilities to the adolescent.

· BE CLEAR THAT DIABETES CARE IS A FAMILY MATTER

Diabetes is not just an individual's disease. It's a family disease. It affects family activities, routines, demands, worries, and emergencies. That's why, no matter what the adolescent's age, effective diabetes care requires that the young person and his family work together as a team. Everyone involved has the same goals—although it may often appear otherwise. This goal is a happy, healthy young adult. This goal can be reached if, and only if, everyone makes diabetes care a partnership. The guidelines that follow describe how to forge such a partnership. These guidelines can also be helpful to parents involved in helping a young person manage his or her diabetes. See Chapter 5 for more on the family's role in diabetes care.

MAKE SURE THAT BLOOD GLUCOSE GOALS ARE REALISTIC

Perfect blood glucose control is an impossible dream. The intensive treatment group of the Diabetes Control and Complications Trial (DCCT), highly motivated as they were and with state-of-the-art professional care, were unable, as a group, to achieve normoglycemia. In fact, only 20% of the group ever achieved a normal HbA_{1c} reading during the course of the trial, and only 5% maintained normal HbA_{1c} levels throughout the study. Among the teenagers who participated in the DCCT, the proportion who achieved normal HbA_{1c} levels was even lower.

Difficult as it is to achieve at any age, normoglycemia is probably uniquely unachievable during adolescence. The physiological changes of this period, which are associated with insulin resistance in both diabetic and nondiabetic teenagers, contribute to blood glucose instability. Combined with the need to test one's wings, which often means less attention to diabetes care, blood glucose control during adolescence is often particularly rocky.

Pushing adolescents and their parents to achieve blood glucose goals that are beyond their reach can actually contribute to poorer glycemic control, since it may lead to feelings of hopelessness and to reduced motivation for self-care.

HELP TEENS AND THEIR PARENTS DEAL WITH FEELINGS

Living with diabetes makes life more stressful, so patients and their parents are bound to feel frustrated, scared, and angry, at least from time to time. When they do, they need a constructive way to let out the feelings. It helps to make clear to them that it's often the diabetes they are upset with, and not each other. Helping patients focus their anger (or other upset feelings) on the diabetes puts teens and their parents on the same side of the fence, and that is a must if they want to get anywhere in their efforts to live successfully with diabetes.

Feeling bad about diabetes is natural, normal, even inevitable. Providers and parents often find it hard to hear a teen talk about how much he hates diabetes, because they don't know what to do about the feelings. They think they have to do something, that they have to somehow protect the child from the pain. But when it comes to feelings, the best thing any caring adult can do, in fact the only thing an adult can do, is to listen to the adolescent and to sympathize with him or her. A relationship based on the teenager's understanding that someone else appreciates how difficult life with diabetes can be is the foundation for working together to help the teenager effectively manage his or her diabetes.

ASK GOOD QUESTIONS

Good questions are the most powerful tool for helping a teenager grow up healthy and happy. Asking good questions is the foundation for an adolescent-clinician-parent diabetes care partnership. Some of the questions to ask are unique to a particular patient and his or her family, while others are common to many families who live with diabetes. Among the latter are questions such as, "What's the hardest thing for you right now about managing your diabetes?," "Is there anything I can do to help?," "What do you think we should do about this problem?" All these questions, and the discussion they engender, are open-ended invitations to the patient to learn to manage his or her diabetes. While there is no guarantee that asking these questions will result in an immediate improvement in patients' self-care and glycemic control, this approach is the only one with a realistic chance of achieving those results over time.

When it comes to good questions, tone and timing are crucial. Parents are especially prone to asking judgmental questions, ones to which they already know (or think they know) the answer. Help parents avoid questions such as, "What did you eat?" (when the adolescent has high blood glucose). When the adolescent's parents ask questions, encourage them to ask questions designed to open up communication with the teenager, to provide information, and to help the teenager take better care of himself or herself. See Chapter 17 for more on the importance of effective questioning.

FOCUS ON SUCCESSES

One of the most important and useful questions to ask is this: "How come *that* worked so well?" There will be times when a problem situation goes more smoothly than usual, and figuring out what helped can be tremendously beneficial. Let's say a teenager usually finds it hard to limit herself to the amount she's supposed to eat when out with friends. Then for a while, she's able to stay on her meal plan. Understanding what made this period different from all others provides invaluable information. Maybe the teen was getting more support from her friends, maybe she was less hungry than usual, or maybe she just didn't feel like fighting with her mother. Whatever the reason, and the reason will be different for different teens, puzzling out what made things work better will help the teen improve self-control. And it will help her learn in the best possible way, by focusing on her successes rather than her failures.

RECOGNIZE THAT NO ONE CAN CONTROL THE ADOLESCENT'S BLOOD GLUCOSE BUT THE ADOLESCENT

Accept the fact, and help parents realize that the clinician's job and their job is *not* to control the adolescent's blood glucose levels, but to help him learn to control them himself. Doing this means being clear about the difference between pushing and supporting.

Supporting a teenager means helping him reach a goal *he* has chosen; pushing a teenager means trying to get him to do something *you* have chosen. No matter how laudable the goal that is being pushed, when pushed, a child is very likely to resist. We aren't suggesting that clinicians let patients make diabetes management decisions completely on their own, but we are suggesting that clinicians let them participate, and even take the lead, in making these decisions.

Taking this approach can be hard for clinicians and for parents, as well. They fear the adolescent will not do the right thing when it comes to diabetes care. And the teen probably won't, all of the time. But the teen will much of the time, if the clinician and parents work with him as he learns the lessons he needs to learn, and as the responsibility for his care is gradually shifted to him.

If this approach makes clinicians uncomfortable, it may help to keep in mind an indisputable fact: if a teenager doesn't "buy in" to the diabetes-care plan that others think he should follow, he will use his veto power anyway. Seeing patients exercise this veto power is probably a daily experience for most diabetes care providers. Helping patients learn to make their own decisions, with providers and parents there to help them, is really the only workable approach. It is also important to keep in mind that this does not contradict the earlier suggestion concerning the need to cooperate in self-care rather than thrusting all responsibility on the teenager. The key to success is working with the adolescent while recognizing the young person's veto power in the process.

BE SPECIFIC

When working with an adolescent toward diabetes treatment goals, the more specifically his problems, vulnerabilities, strengths, and successes are defined, the easier life will be. Rita was a high school senior who had been diagnosed with diabetes at the age of 7 and had managed it well. Suddenly, she started running really high blood glucose levels. It turned out that Rita was going to the mall every night after dinner and hanging out with her friends. One of their favorite activities, other than talking, was eating. Rita joined in, and by the time she got home, her blood glucose was very high. For some reason, at this point, Rita told herself that it was "too late" to do anything about the hyperglycemia. The fact that Rita could acknowledge she had a problem and that she could be so specific in describing it was an invaluable step toward finding a solution.

Naturally, the solution had to be equally specific, and Rita was very clear that she *would not* 1) stop going to the mall, 2) stop eating when she went to the mall, 3) carry her insulin with her to the mall, and 4) take an extra shot when she got home. Though in a way Rita was being difficult, in another way, she was being helpful, because she was making it clear what would not work. After offering a few suggestions and having Rita veto them, her physician came up with a suggestion she was willing to try: taking a syringe with 4 units of Regular insulin in it with her to the mall in her purse. Rita said she would go to the bathroom right before she ate and give herself whatever part of the 4 units she felt she needed to cover the food she had ordered. This worked for her because she could do it so quickly.

When trying to work toward specific solutions with patients, keep this image in mind: help a patient describe a problem (or a solution) so specifically that a movie could be made of it. Getting that specific sometimes takes time and work. Often, it involves asking deeper and deeper questions about a situation, seeking to discover what's really going on, like solving a mystery. Approaching this effort in this spirit might help. Think about the energy a typical teenager is willing to put out to do things that really interest him. Wouldn't it be wonderful if he could tap that energy and enthusiasm in his efforts to learn to manage his diabetes?

MAINTAIN CONTACT

It's important to check in regularly with adolescent patients to see how they are doing. This can be difficult, given the busy schedules most clinicians maintain, but any contact can be helpful. Think about what's available, even if it's only a couple of extra minutes each time the teenager comes in. Ask her about any new problems that might have come up, about any successes she's had managing her diabetes, and about anything noticeable that needs discussion. When time is limited, try to focus on whatever issue is of greatest concern to the adolescent.

It's also essential that patients' parents do all they can to maintain contact with their children. Some families have regularly scheduled diabetes family meetings when everyone gets to say anything they want about how things have been going since the last meeting. This can be a good opportunity to deal with small problems before they become big ones. The key to success with these meetings is maintaining an attitude of cooperation.

SUPPORT PROBLEM-SOLVING SKILLS

Let patients know they can do anything they set their minds to, but that achieving their goals may require refined problem-solving skills. A teenager who had only a few days earlier begun using an insulin pump was planning to go out to dinner with his father. The meal was a special occasion, and the young man had talked his father into letting him order anything he wanted. Unfortunately, his predinner blood glucose level was 350 mg/dl. Taking a chance on his son's budding diabetes problem-solving skills, and hoping to strengthen them, the father agreed to stick with the agreement on the condition that the young man think really hard about how much insulin he needed to take to cover the meal and that he test his blood 2 hours and 4 hours after dinner. Even after a big dinner, the results of these tests were 220 mg/dl and 150 mg/dl. The boy explained his success: "I calculated how much carbohydrate was in each thing I ate, and I used the formula I was taught to figure the amount of insulin I needed. I really wanted that food, and I really didn't want to feel sick later, so I worked hard to get the insulin right."

Support problem-solving by asking patients questions: "What do you need to do so you can safely do whatever it is you want to do?" If something went wrong in managing his diabetes, ask what lesson he learned that he could apply next time he is in a similar situation. And if something went *right*, the same question is also appropriate. Try to get the patient's parents to facilitate this kind of problem-solving, too.

HELP BUILD EMOTIONAL STRENGTH

Dealing effectively with diabetes requires emotional strength as well as problem-solving skills. We've found that the fundamental elements of this emotional strength are love, faith, and humor. Clinicians would do well to foster these qualities in themselves and their patients' parents, and nurture them in their teenage patients.

It is said that love conquers all, and when it comes to coping with the stress of life with diabetes, this may well be true. Love gives us confidence, and it just plain feels wonderful. Make sure the hassles and aggravations of daily life with diabetes don't prevent patients and their families from enjoying, appreciating, and loving each other.

Optimism is another bulwark against the stresses and strains of daily life with diabetes. Draw upon any source of optimism and help patients and their families do the same. Think of the improvements being made in diabetes care. Think about successes with patients. Think about the fortitude and creativity many patients display. Forty years ago, a 13-year-old became the first person in her family to be diagnosed with diabetes. When the girl asked her mother what having diabetes would mean for them, her mother responded, "It means we will learn to eat better than we have ever eaten before, we will all be healthier than we ever were before, and we will all learn to love each other more than we ever did before."

Humor is wonderful. Along with faith, it's the closest thing to magic in the world. How often has someone said, "I don't know how I would have made it if it hadn't been for my sense of humor?" Humor helps keep things in perspective; it protects people from feeling overwhelmed. If clinicians can help patients and their families apply humor to their lives with diabetes, they will be providing them a real service.

The essence of humor is taking a bad situation and exaggerating its awfulness to the point it is so ridiculous it becomes funny. Fortunately or unfortunately, life with diabetes presents us with plenty of material for humor. Try to find some humor in patients' daily experiences and see what can be made of it.

GET HELP

There will be times when diabetes is too much for a young person to handle alone, even with the help and support of a health-care team and family. When this is true, try to direct the patient to the help he or she needs. This might mean referral for specialized mental health services. Refer to other chapters in this book for criteria to use in deciding if referral to a mental health professional is warranted and for suggestions about making referrals in a way that is helpful and constructive rather than blaming and stigmatizing, as perceived by the adolescent and parents. Getting help can also mean helping the patient and his or her family find support groups, such as those available in many areas under the auspices of the American Diabetes Association or Juvenile Diabetes Foundation, or hospitals and other organizations, as well.

CONCLUSION

Working with adolescents who have diabetes can be uniquely challenging. But if clinicians work wisely with patients and their parents, facilitating the process by which young people learn to manage their disease, their work can be uniquely rewarding, as well.

BIBLIOGRAPHY

Amiel SA, Sherwin RS, Simonson DC, Lauritano AA, Tamborlane WV: Impaired glucose tolerance in puberty: a contributing factor to poor glycemic control in adolescents with diabetes. *N Engl J Med* 315:215–219, 1986

Anderson BJ: The home team advantage. *Diabetes Self-Management* 11:55–59, 1994

Rubin RR, Biermann J, Toohey B: *Psyching Out Diabetes.* Los Angeles, Lowell House, 1992

Solowiegcyzk J, Baker L: Being an adolescent with diabetes. *Diabetes Care* 1:124–125, 1978

Wysocki T, Taylor A, Hough B, Linscheid T, Yeates K, Naglieri J: Deviation from developmentally appropriate self-care autonomy. *Diabetes Self-Care* 19:119–125, 1996

Improving Diabetes Control in Adolescents With Type I Diabetes

3

Joseph I. Wolfsdorf, MB, BCh

INTRODUCTION

Optimal treatment of diabetes during puberty is necessary to ensure normal growth and secondary sexual development and to prevent the appearance or slow the progression of diabetic microvascular complications. The Diabetes Control and Complications Trial (DCCT) demonstrated that both the direction and magnitude of the beneficial effects of intensive therapy in adolescents were similar to those observed in adults. Intensive therapy for achieving glycemic control is considered the new standard of care for type I diabetes. The mandate for all clinicians is to help adolescent patients lower blood glucose levels to normal or as near to normal as possible. Developmental considerations and the endocrinologic effects of puberty conspire to make this a daunting task.

LESSONS FROM THE DCCT

Of the 1,441 subjects who participated in the DCCT, 13.5% were adolescents (13 to 17 years old at the time of enrollment) who were followed for a mean of 7.4 years. At baseline, the mean hemoglobin A1c (HbA$_{1c}$) in the adolescent cohort was ~9.5% (upper limit of normal is 6.05%), whereas the adult cohort started with a mean HbA$_{1c}$ of ~8.5%. With institution of intensive diabetes therapy, mean HbA$_{1c}$ levels of both the adult and adolescent cohorts decreased by about 2 percent-

TABLE 1. *Mean HbA$_{1c}$ Levels of Adolescents Compared With Adults in the DCCT*

Treatment	Adolescents (%)	Adults (%)
Intensive	8.06 ± 0.13	7.12 ± 0.03
Conventional	9.76 ± 0.12	9.02 ± 0.05
Difference (intensive vs. conventional)	1.70 ± 0.18	1.90 ± 0.06

Data are means ± SE. Adapted from DCCT Research Group: Effect of intensive diabetes treatment on the development and progression of long-term complications in adolescents with insulin-dependent diabetes mellitus: Diabetes Control and Complications Trial. *J Pediatr* 125:177–188, 1994

age points. By the end of the first year of the study, it was already evident that the adolescent cohort was unable to lower blood glucose and HbA$_{1c}$ to the same levels achieved by the adult cohort. This difference between adolescents and adults, noted early in the course of the study, persisted for the duration. In a select patient population receiving "state-of-the-art" diabetes care with all the necessary resources at their disposal, <2% of adolescents maintained HbA$_{1c}$ levels ≤6.05%, and only 29% were able to achieve the study target of ≤6.05% at least once in the course of the study. Mean HbA$_{1c}$ levels of adolescents are compared with those of adults in Table 1. Expectations for HbA$_{1c}$ levels for adolescent patients compared with adult patients must reflect these realistic limitations.

ADOLESCENT DEVELOPMENTAL CONSIDERATIONS

Treatment of type I diabetes in children and adolescents occurs on a background of physical, cognitive, and emotional growth and development. Until maturity is attained, developmental issues frequently influence the health-care team's efforts to manage diabetes. Despite the challenges, patiently, but persistently, help the patient to manage his or her diabetes as well as possible, mindful of the fact that the ideal goals of therapy currently may not be achievable in an individual patient.

ENDOCRINOLOGIC EFFECTS OF PUBERTY

Glycemic control often deteriorates with the onset of puberty. This is usually attributed to adolescents' poor compliance with diet and insulin administration. But behavioral and psychosocial issues are not the only factors that affect blood glucose control during this stage of development. Endocrinologic changes of puberty significantly contribute to the deterioration in glycemic control.

- Insulin resistance normally occurs during puberty; and the adverse effects of both puberty and diabetes on insulin action contribute to difficulty achieving optimal glycemic control in adolescents.
- During puberty, physiological insulin resistance results in an increase in the daily insulin requirement. As much as 1.5 U/kg/day may be necessary to achieve optimal glycemic control.
- Diurnal variation in insulin requirements, which reach a nadir between midnight and 3 A.M. and increase from 5 to 9 A.M. (the dawn phenomenon), is often more pronounced during puberty.
- During the period of accelerated growth, both nutritional and insulin requirements markedly increase. To ensure the best possible metabolic control, schedule follow-up visits for medical supervision at least once every 3 months until completion of growth. These visits provide an opportunity to review the insulin regimen to determine if insulin doses need to be adjusted and to make necessary changes in the meal plan.

INSULIN REGIMENS

Many patients can achieve acceptable blood glucose control with conventional insulin therapy (defined as two daily doses, one before breakfast and one before supper, of a mixture of regular and intermediate-acting insulins), provided they are willing to adhere to a rigid schedule of insulin administration, meals, and snacks. Few adolescents will tolerate such an imposition on their lifestyles, but many are willing to accept a regimen of more frequent insulin administration (either with a conventional syringe or an insulin pen device) that permits greater flexibility of meal times and lifestyle in general.

Successful use of any multiple-dose regimen requires extensive self-management training to enable the youth to interpret self-monitoring of blood glucose (SMBG) data, to adjust timing of insulin injections and doses, and to make appropriate food selections. **The goal is to equip the adolescent patient with problem-solving skills to cope with unexpected situations and unplanned events typical of the adolescent lifestyle**; for example, additional, late, or omitted meals, "pickup" games, travel to events away from home, participation in competitive sports, and variable sleep times.

- After the honeymoon or remission period, which frequently begins immediately after diagnosis and extends for 3 to 12 months or longer, optimal delivery of insulin requires multiple doses of insulin.
- If an adolescent patient is not already using a multiple-dose insulin (MDI) regimen, encourage him or her to use a three-dose regimen: a mixed dose (regular and intermediate-acting insulins) before breakfast, regular insulin before the evening meal, and intermediate-acting insulin (with or without regular insulin) delayed until bedtime.
- Regimens in which intermediate-acting insulin is given before the evening meal do not permit ideal insulin delivery overnight. Too much insulin is provided in the early part of the night, which may cause symptomatic or asymptomatic hypoglycemia between 11 P.M. and 4 A.M.; whereas insufficient insulin action before breakfast results in high fasting and post-breakfast blood glucose concentrations.
- For those willing and able to take regular insulin before lunch at school or before a large after-school snack, a fourth dose may be the best approach to prevent hyperglycemia in the late afternoon. This is not always necessary, and for the youth unwilling to use a four-dose regimen, a mixed dose of insulin before breakfast can achieve excellent blood glucose control if the calorie content of the midday meal is not excessive.

NUTRITION

- Attention must be paid to the timing and content of meals in order to match food intake with the availability of injected insulin.

- The main aim of nutritional counseling is to encourage the patient to use a meal plan that fits his or her lifestyle, promotes optimal compliance, and advances the goals of management.
- In the DCCT, adherence to a prescribed meal plan and adjusting food and/or insulin in response to hyperglycemia were associated with significantly lower (0.25 to 1.0%) levels of HbA_{1c}. Adjusting the insulin dose for meal size and content and consistent consumption of an evening snack were also associated with lower levels of HbA_{1c}. These findings underscore the importance of nutritional counseling to enhance the patient's ability to adjust food intake to match available insulin.
- From the time of diagnosis and at follow-up visits, instruct the patient on the principles of nutritional management of diabetes and formulate an individualized meal plan that minimizes postprandial hyperglycemia and hypoglycemia between meals.
- Teach patients how to respond to high blood glucose levels; for example, to take supplemental regular insulin and to wait 45 to 60 minutes after injecting insulin before eating.
- The process of nutrition education is staged; it begins with "survival" information and gradually progresses to more advanced topics: using food exchanges, counting carbohydrates, reading food labels, and selecting from restaurant menus.

EXERCISE

- Encourage teenagers with diabetes to participate in sports and to exercise regularly throughout the year. In addition to normalizing the child's life and helping to form a positive self-image, exercise promotes good health practices, facilitates weight control, and may improve glycemic control by decreasing the physiological insulin resistance of puberty. Adolescents with type I diabetes who maintain a high level of physical fitness are relatively less insulin resistant.
- Exercise acutely lowers the blood glucose concentration by increasing its rate of utilization. Overall glucose utilization depends on the intensity and duration of physical activity and the concurrent serum level of insulin. Teach teenagers strategies to prevent exercise-related hypoglycemia. Ideally, when starting a new ex-

ercise program, have teenagers measure blood glucose before, during, and after exercise so that rational adjustments can be made to the insulin dose, meals, and snacks.

- In the absence of SMBG data, have teenagers cover unplanned physical activity with a snack before and, if the exercise is prolonged, during the activity. A useful rule of thumb is to provide 15 grams of carbohydrate (one Starch or Fruit Exchange) for every 30 to 60 minutes of vigorous physical activity.
- Advise youth who participate in organized sports to reduce the dose of the insulin that is most active during the period of sustained physical activity. The precise amount of such reductions has to be determined by measuring blood glucose levels before and after exercise. These reductions are generally in the range of 10 to 30% of the usual insulin dose.
- Exercising the limb into which insulin has been injected accelerates its rate of absorption; therefore, have patients give the insulin injection preceding planned exercise in a site where absorption is least likely to be affected by exercise.
- After strenuous exercise in the afternoon or evening, have patients take a 10 to 20% reduction in the presupper and/or bedtime dose of intermediate-acting insulin, together with a larger bedtime snack, to reduce the risk of nocturnal or early-morning hypoglycemia from the lag effect of exercise.
- Make sure the youth is aware that ketonuria is a reason not to exercise, because vigorous exercise under these circumstances can aggravate hyperglycemia and ketoacid production.

MONITORING DIABETES CONTROL

- SMBG data are the cornerstone of intensive diabetes management.
- Frequent SMBG is essential to manage intercurrent illness and prevent ketoacidosis. Have the patient test his or her urine for the presence of ketones whenever sick and when the level of blood glucose exceeds 250 mg/dl.
- Check on the ability of the patient to obtain accurate SMBG results by comparing results obtained with his or her meter with simultaneous blood glucose measurements on a laboratory instrument.

- Encourage patients to measure blood glucose levels before each meal and at bedtime. If this is impractical or intolerable, blood glucose measurements before each dose of insulin and before lunch and at bedtime at least twice each week is an acceptable alternative. For patients unwilling to perform regular SMBG, a period of intensive monitoring (before each meal, at bedtime, and between 2 and 4 A.M.) for several consecutive days before an office visit may provide sufficient information to confirm satisfactory glycemic control or reveal a blood glucose pattern that calls for simple modifications of the insulin regimen. Obviously, such a patient is not a candidate for intensive diabetes management.
- Teenagers frequently fabricate blood glucose measurements because of pressure from their family members and physicians to produce "good" results. This behavior can be minimized if parents and physicians avoid being judgmental when reviewing SMBG data with the patient.
- Instructing patients to measure blood glucose levels without teaching them how to interpret the data is unlikely to improve diabetes control. Rather than use the data as the patient's "diabetes report card," as is all too often done, use the information as an opportunity to instruct and educate the patient in self-management skills. This includes, but is not limited to, how to: analyze and interpret the numbers, use insulin dosage algorithms to select and adjust doses of insulin, make appropriate food choices, and plan exercise.
- Have an HbA_{1c} test done every 3 months to provide a measure of average glycemia in the intervals between office visits.

BIOCHEMICAL GOALS OF THERAPY

The goal of treatment is to maintain blood glucose levels as close to normal as possible while minimizing the occurrence of hypoglycemia. The DCCT found that any reduction in HbA_{1c} level was rewarded by a reduction in the risk of microvascular complications. However, the DCCT also demonstrated that even with intensive methods of treatment and unlimited access to expert medical advice and supervision, it is extremely difficult to achieve the goal of near-normal HbA_{1c} levels in adolescents with type I diabetes.

HYPOGLYCEMIA

Hypoglycemia is the principal adverse effect of intensive diabetes management and can be a major obstacle to achieving and maintaining tight glycemic control. Fear of hypoglycemia is an important determinant of patients' personal goals for glycemic control. In the DCCT, both intensively managed adults and adolescents had three times as many episodes of severe hypoglycemia as their conventionally treated peers. The overall incidence of severe hypoglycemia was even higher in adolescents than in adults, 86 vs. 57 events per 100 patient-years. However, the reduction in risk of microvascular and neurologic complications in adolescents outweighs the increased risk of severe hypoglycemia.

Be mindful of adolescent patients' vulnerability to hypoglycemia. Teach patients how to anticipate and prevent hypoglycemia and to treat it promptly without causing hyperglycemia. Begin treatment with 15 grams of glucose (preferably in the form of glucose tablets); repeat the dose if the blood glucose level has not risen after 20 minutes. Practical guidelines for reducing the risk of hypoglycemia appear in Chapters 9 and 10 of this book.

RESPONSIBILITY FOR DIABETES CARE

Cognitive Maturity

The ability of an adolescent with type I diabetes to successfully assume primary responsibility for his or her diabetes care is related to age and the individual's level of cognitive maturity. Intensive management of type I diabetes requires considerable patient participation in self-care and day-to-day decision-making. Indeed, the patient with diabetes has to learn to become his or her own health-care provider.

Technical mastery of self-care skills and a thorough knowledge of the disease and its treatment are essential to assuming this role. The willingness and the ability to perform the numerous tasks required to safely achieve desirable blood glucose control depend substantially on the individual's level of cognitive maturity. Age alone must not determine the appropriate time to transfer responsibility for self-care from parents to their adolescent child. The process of transfer should be gradual, accomplished over years, with decreasing parental supervision as the adolescent consistently demonstrates the ability to care competently for himself or herself without deterioration of blood glucose control.

Family Functioning

Adolescents are dependent on their parents for material as well as emotional support and guidance. The functioning of the family system, therefore, has a major influence on the adolescent patient's diabetes care behavior and adherence to the regimen (see Chapter 5). Intensive management can be realistically and safely applied to the care of a youth with diabetes only if the family has the requisite emotional and economic resources. The cost of intensive therapy is approximately twice that of conventional therapy. The ability and willingness of a family to assume any additional expenses they must bear may be an important factor limiting the clinician's ability to intensify a patient's management.

The Adherence Problem

Adherence to a complex, demanding, intensive diabetes regimen requires lifelong changes in behavior and involves repeated daily performance of several unpleasant tasks: injections, testing, dietary modifications, and exercise routines. Only a tiny minority of patients comply with all the elements necessary for optimal glycemic control. Poor adherence to the prescribed regimen, therefore, is a major impediment to maintaining optimal health of individuals with diabetes. It is now clear that readmission for diabetic ketoacidosis is usually due to major deviations from recommended therapy and, most importantly, to missed insulin injections.

It is important to recognize the existence and prevalence of mismanagement and candidly and nonjudgmentally discuss these behaviors with patients and their families.

- Make concrete strategies for avoiding or minimizing mismanagement a standard part of diabetes education for all patients and their families. Address the patient's goals and earn his or her trust by being willing to compromise. Recommend small changes, and implement them at a rate that the patient can tolerate.

- Encourage parents to play an active role in their adolescents' diabetes care. This notion may run counter to the conventional wisdom of allowing adolescents to assume responsibility for their own management, but research and clinical experience reveal that increased parental involvement and supervision are effective in decreasing nonadherence, preventing ketoacidosis, and improving glycemic control in teenagers.
- Sharing the burden of care with family members is especially important when the adolescent patient is not achieving the goals of therapy. Determine the degree of parental involvement by the adolescent's success in self-management.

CONCLUSION

Although improving diabetes control in adolescents is an arduous task for patients, families, and clinicians alike, one cannot shrink from the challenge. Because any sustained reduction in the level of glycosylated hemoglobin lowers the risk of diabetic microvascular and neuropathic complications, make every effort to prevent deterioration of glycemic control during the adolescent years.

BIBLIOGRAPHY

Amiel S, Sherwin R, Simonson D, Lauritano A, Tamborlane W: Impaired insulin action in puberty: a contributing factor to poor glycemic control in adolescents with diabetes. *N Engl J Med* 31:215–219, 1986

Connell J, Thomas-Dobersen D: Nutritional management of children and adolescents with insulin-dependent diabetes mellitus: a review by the diabetes care and education dietetic practice group. *J Am Diet Assoc* 91:1556–1564, 1991

DCCT Research Group: Diabetes Control and Complications Trial (DCCT): the effect of intensive treatment of diabetes on the development and progression of long-term complications in insulin-dependent diabetes mellitus. *N Engl J Med* 329:977–986, 1993

DCCT Research Group: Effect of intensive diabetes treatment on the development and progression of long-term complications in adolescents with insulin-dependent diabetes mellitus: Diabetes Control and Complications Trial. *J Pediatr* 125:177–188, 1994

Delahanty L, Halford B: The role of diet behaviors in achieving glycemic control in intensively treated patients in the Diabetes Control and Complications Trial. *Diabetes Care* 16:1453–1458, 1993

Krolewski A, Laffel L, Krolewski M, Quinn M, Warram J: Glycosylated hemoglobin and the risk of microalbuminuria in patients with insulin-dependent diabetes mellitus. *N Engl J Med* 332:1251–1255, 1995

Schmidt L, Colby P, Kwong C: Practical nutritional guidelines to reduce the risk of hypoglycemia in patients treated with insulin. *Clin Diabetes* 3:46–48, 1995

Weir G, Nathan D, Singer D: Standards of care for diabetes. *Diabetes Care* 17:1514–1522, 1994

Caring for Elderly Patients With Diabetes | 4

John F. Zrebiec, MSW

INTRODUCTION

Diabetes requires active, daily patient participation to maintain metabolic control. The need for self-care behaviors does not diminish with age. In fact, older adults face special challenges because of the physical, social, functional, and psychological changes that may be imposed by the aging process, the complications from diabetes, and the presence of multiple chronic illnesses. This chapter focuses on several psychological principles and behavioral strategies for successful management of the elderly patient.

UNDERSTAND THE NORMAL DEVELOPMENTAL TASKS OF AGING

Aging is a normal phase of life and not a pathological development. For most people, aging does not mean increasing depression or dementia, but neither are these "golden years" often spent in carefree living, fishing, and baking cookies for the grandchildren. The transition to retirement confronts people with challenges to their intellectual vitality, social life, and sense of worth. The primary developmental tasks are to establish new roles and activities, develop compassion toward parents and children, tolerate the physical and cognitive changes of the aging process, accept the past, and discover a meaningful purpose for the remainder of life.

Certain life crises are a normal part of aging. Loss is the most important and difficult occurrence, and grief is the most common experience as a person loses spouse, family, and friends. Physical illness is the other major hurdle that faces the elderly. The ubiquitous preoccupation with the body and its functions is a normal consequence of aging, with its increasing probability of illness, hospitalization, surgery, pain, and disability. The possibility for developing complications from diabetes adds to this predictable challenge to remaining independent and productive.

For the clinician, it is important to consider the tasks that lie ahead for the patient, the capacity that is available to master those tasks, and the kind of help that is needed.

UNDERSTAND THE CLINICIAN'S PERSPECTIVE ON AGING

Clinician's attitudes toward elderly patients affect the care that these patients receive. Difficulty in empathizing with older patients commonly occurs because the clinician

- Believes that old people cannot change or are too old to want to change, therefore making suggestions useless.
- Views diabetes as simply part of the aging process and, therefore, not very serious.
- Lets the patient's fears stimulate his or her own fears of old age, death, or the future.
- Lets the patient's conflicts trigger thoughts of his or her own personal conflicts.
- Tends to infantilize the older person because he or she seems weak or vulnerable.

To Avoid These Problems

1. Stay alert to inappropriate, exaggerated, ambivalent, erratic, or tenacious feelings toward the patient.
2. Have a personal support system for discussion of feelings.
3. Share care responsibilities with the rest of the team.
4. Maintain an appropriate professional distance.

UNDERSTAND THE PATIENT'S PERSPECTIVE ON AGING

While elderly people are more likely to accept diabetes as part of the aging process, they are also more likely to perceive diabetes as less serious and, therefore, in less need of careful management. In addition, many older adults have other chronic illnesses that cause more suffering and require more attention. Basically, a person's perception about diabetes is an important factor in determining adherence. These perceptions often include beliefs about cause, seriousness, consequences, sense of control, and treatment effectiveness. One recent study found that beliefs about the effectiveness of treatment and the degree of satisfaction with medical care were the factors most predictive of dietary intake and physical activity. These beliefs about treatment, in themselves, result from a mixture of family attitudes about diabetes, past experiences with medical care, subjective distress due to complications or blood glucose results, and self-esteem.

The key point is that older people want to have their medical concerns listened to and taken seriously. It is imperative to ask patients about how diabetes affects their life and what parts of diabetes care are difficult.

UNDERSTAND THE ROLE OF FUNCTIONAL STATUS

It is important to understand the elderly patient's functional status, that is, how the patient functions in activities of everyday living, like fastening buttons or walking stairs. In fact, the patient's functional skills may be of more immediate importance than his or her metabolic status. Functional assessment is also crucial because practical medical management and realistic treatment goals rest upon an understanding of the capabilities of the older patient. A medical history may be helpful, but observation is key. For example, impaired hearing and vision can interfere with effective communication and the ability to understand educational directions or medical recommendations. Techniques such as eliminating extraneous noises, speaking slowly and in deep tones while facing the patient, writing questions in large print, and providing adequate lighting can be helpful. It is important to notice whether the patient:

1. Can see well enough to measure insulin, do blood glucose monitoring, and inspect his or her feet.
2. Can hear well enough to understand medical recommendations.
3. Is physically fit enough to climb stairs, handle a wheelchair, get on the exam table, get out of bed, open pill bottles, shop, cook, bathe and dress, or comply with exercise prescriptions to walk, swim, or bicycle.
4. Is alert and oriented enough to remember medication regimens, dietary restrictions, and follow-up appointments.

It is important to ask specific questions about symptoms and diabetes management, because elderly patients tend to underreport details if they

• Are ashamed, misguided, or uneducated about diabetes.
• Fear illness.
• Want to please the clinician.
• Expect illness as a normal part of aging.

For example, without detailed questioning, older people might never mention problems with sexual function because they are embarrassed, assume it is a consequence of aging, or are unaware of the effects of neuropathy.

Elderly patients with multiple complaints can frustrate the clinician who is trying to figure out the causes. These complaints, however, can be deceiving. Somatic complaints may be representations of underlying emotional distress in addition to symptoms of illness. Similarly, reports of physical illness may be exaggerated by emotional distress. In sorting out these complex dynamics, there is no substitute for spending time getting to know the patient. Yet, it is often not realistic to gather all the essential information in one long appointment that exhausts both the patient and the clinician. Shorter appointments with briefer agendas, spread over a few sessions, may prove more effective in gathering information without pressuring the older person.

IDENTIFY BARRIERS TO SELF-CARE

The lack of basic economic resources can have a tremendous impact on the older person. It can mean that the medical attention and supplies needed for diabetes care become secondary to the need for food, clothing, and shelter. For example, adequate nutrition may be more important than blood glucose monitoring. The clinician needs to carefully assess income, housing, home care, resources for food, clothing, transportation, utilities, personal care and recreation, medical insurance, legal factors, and, of course, family support of patients. The clinician may need to be an advocate for the older person by not only taking responsibility for assessing the resources available but also actually connecting the patient with formal services. For example, a patient neither filled her prescriptions for metformin nor kept all her medical appointments because she did not have a telephone or transportation. The doctor called in her prescriptions to the pharmacy and arranged for delivery, while the social worker arranged for free transportation to clinic appointments. These strategies do require frequent, time-consuming health provider involvement with the patient, but the payoff in adherence to treatment recommendations is worth the effort.

SET SMALL, REALISTIC GOALS

Patients are very likely aware of their poor habits that cause blood glucose problems. This awareness often makes them feel guilty and ashamed, and it does not help to blame patients or expect them to have more self-discipline. They have already had a lifetime in which to change habits, and it may now be a formidable task to ask someone to change a lifetime of eating and drinking in a certain way. Remember that adherence to diabetes management is negatively influenced by the duration and extent of behavioral changes required and the complexity of treatment regimens. Few things will undermine motivation and create discouragement quicker than the inability to achieve a goal. Try to appreciate how small interventions can make a major impact on the quality of life.

Make one or two changes at a time. For example, changing one item at breakfast may be a more realistic goal than revamping the person's entire meal plan. Easy armchair aerobics or walking may be more practical than going to a gym.

Many older people are afraid of the change from pills to insulin. Introducing the change through small steps may help alleviate their fears. Have the person stay on oral agents while starting to take a small dose of intermediate-acting insulin at bedtime. In this way, the person gets use to handling syringes, finds that the injections are not like the immunizations remembered from youth, sees success and feels better, and is already on a split dose if he or she has to start morning insulin. Another technique is to ask the person to try insulin for 1 month to find out if he or she feels better.

INCLUDE THE FAMILY

A careful assessment of the elderly patient always requires a review of family and social support. In many cases, family members are managers of the diabetes care, monitors of adherence with medical recommendations, and providers of transportation to appointments. Get a description and evaluation of the richness of relationships, the degree of social activity, and the level of diabetes self-management from not only the patient but also the close relatives. Family members can also be asked about the patient's history. The more involved and educated the family is, the easier it will be for them to understand and support the patient in adhering to treatment recommendations. Family meetings in which treatment plans are openly discussed, realistic alternatives are reviewed, and decisions are shared can be very productive. Both research and clinical evidence suggest that family support has a positive impact on diabetes management.

STAY ALERT FOR SIGNS OF DEPRESSION

Depression may be three times more prevalent in people with diabetes than in the general adult population, and depression in the elderly is probably underrecognized and undertreated (see Chapter 15). Depression is often the direct result of escalating complications from diabetes, the demands of management, or the frustrations of erratic blood glucose control. Decreased adherence to treatment, decreased physical activity, and poor glycemic control are, in turn, often the result of depression. Depression often increases alcohol use, which is an important consideration in working with the older person because of its psychological and physical effects. The clinician needs to ask whether the patient thinks (or others have mentioned) that alcohol consumption is a problem.

The diagnosis of depression is not easy. Some drugs, such as blood pressure and heart medications and tranquilizers, can cause depression. Moreover, the symptoms produced by hyperglycemia are often mistaken for depression. The diagnosis gets even more complicated when there is cognitive impairment. The distinction between depression and dementia is crucial, because depression is reversible and often quickly responds to supportive treatment and antidepressant medications.

CONCLUSION

Understanding the psychosocial realities faced by the older person with diabetes is important when designing successful diabetes treatment regimens. This chapter has suggested several strategies for optimizing diabetes management in the elderly patient. Key components of these strategies are the inclusion of the patient's family in both functional assessment and diabetes treatment, and setting practical achievable goals. The underpinnings of this approach rely upon the clinician's understanding of the normal developmental tasks confronting the older person, the psychological and functional challenges superimposed by diabetes, and a nonjudgmental attitude about aging and diabetes control.

BIBLIOGRAPHY

Funnell MM, Merritt JH: The challenge of diabetes and older adults. *Nurs Clin North Am* 28:45-60, 1993

Halter JB, Christensen NJ (Eds.): Diabetes mellitus in elderly people. *Diabetes Care* 13:1–96, 1990

Hampson SE, Glasgow RE, Foster LS: Personal models of diabetes among older adults: relationship to self-management and other variables. *The Diabetes Educator* 21:300–307, 1995

Kane RL, Ouslander J, Abrass IB: *Essentials of Clinical Geriatrics.* New York, McGraw-Hill, 1993

Mooradian AG (Ed.): Diabetes in the elderly. *Diabetes Spectrum* 7:357–383, 1994

Ruggiero L, Clark MM (Eds.): Obesity management in people with diabetes. *Diabetes Spectrum* 5:198–237, 1992

Involving Family Members in Diabetes Treatment

5

Barbara J. Anderson, PhD

INTRODUCTION

Research has taught us that family support is a critical component of successful diabetes management for children, adolescents, and adults. For clinicians faced with caring for more and more patients in less and less time, extending diabetes care to include family members may seem unrealistic. But research indicates that family members can actually make the clinician's job easier and help the patient achieve optimum health and quality of life.

Forging an effective therapeutic alliance with patients' families does take time and effort. Family members do not automatically give the support that patients need. Support must be individually defined for each patient within each family system. Moreover, support is dynamic and changes over time, as the patient and family grow and change.

When the clinician begins to involve family members in diabetes treatment, two general guidelines are important. First, because diabetes affects every facet of family life, the family's ethnic and cultural heritage must be taken into consideration. Second, in families with severely dysfunctional interaction patterns or families in which a member has serious psychiatric problems, successful involvement of the family in diabetes treatment may not be feasible.

In this chapter, four fundamental principles for successfully involving family members in diabetes treatment will be identified; then each will be discussed in detail.

1. Teach the family about diabetes and its treatment, beginning at diagnosis.
2. Listen to and identify diabetes-related feelings of family members. The family's concerns and worries about diabetes need to be addressed, and the family needs to learn that diabetes often brings a full range of feelings (e.g., fear, frustration, guilt, anger, etc.).
3. Teach family members to have realistic and appropriate expectations concerning the patient's medical and behavioral goals.
4. Teach family members how to provide effective support without pushing or controlling the patient, which only serves to undermine the patient's own attempts at healthy diabetes self-care.

PRINCIPLES

Teach the Family About Diabetes and Its Treatment

At the time of diagnosis, encourage patients to bring in their family support person for an educational and getting-acquainted session, which occurs with a medical visit. The support person may be a spouse, a girlfriend or boyfriend, a roommate, a grandparent or sibling of the patient, or any other caregiver of the patient.

For established patients, invite them to bring in a supportive family member at any time. Many patients will not initiate a family meeting on their own. Some patients may state that they do not want help or support from anyone in their family. Encourage these patients to include and educate family members.

Use this session to begin general education about diabetes as a chronic disease with a complex medical treatment regimen. Tell family members about the possible causes of diabetes, changes in the treatment of diabetes over the past 20 years, and the impact of diabetes on many dimensions of family life—daily routines, finances, celebrations, and meal schedules.

Find out what the family believes or knows about diabetes. In order to learn about family beliefs about diabetes, ask a question such as "Have any of your friends or other relatives had diabetes or diabetes complications?"

Listen to the Family's Feelings About Diabetes and Their Current Concerns About the Patient

Listening to the family's concerns about diabetes is not a recommendation to do family therapy, but rather family education. It is not critical to have a solution or answer for every feeling voiced by the patient's spouse or parent. What is important is that feelings are voiced and concerns are raised, and that feelings based on mistaken beliefs are exposed as early in the course of the disease as possible. Diabetes normally brings into families a range of complex feelings, such as the following:

Guilt. Feelings of guilt are often a burden to a parent or grandparent who believes that because diabetes is in his or her family, he or she is solely responsible for the diabetes. It is important to explain that no one gene causes diabetes, and that no one side of the family is responsible for diabetes. State clearly that there are still many unanswered question about the causes of diabetes, but that current thinking is that diabetes comes from both sides of the family and is caused by environmental as well as genetic factors.

Blame. Blame can be crippling. It can prevent many patients from ever getting fully involved in their own diabetes self-care. In overweight patients with type II diabetes, it is a common mistake for family members to believe that overeating and excessive weight gain alone caused the diabetes. It is important to explain that scientists do not yet know all of the risk factors for type I or type II diabetes and are not yet able to prevent it.

Financial concerns. Family members sometimes worry about the financial burden of diabetes supplies as well as about health and life insurance coverage for the patient. Diabetes does bring extra expenses into the family. Therefore, health insurance coverage is critical for people with diabetes. When concerns arise about financial and health insurance issues, they are often handled most effectively by referral to a skilled medical social worker. Local chapters of the American Diabetes Association and Juvenile Diabetes Foundation can sometimes help in finding the best buys in diabetes supplies at a local level.

Loss of a "normal lifestyle." Many family members worry that life will never again seem normal. Ask family members to identify their major concerns. Then begin to help the family address these concerns. Contact with a support group or with other families who have managed successfully may help to communicate that after a period of adjustment, most families achieve a *new* normal lifestyle.

Fears. Family members are frequently afraid of the long-term complications of diabetes. For these families, it is important to reassure them that all their efforts to help the patient maintain good blood glucose control are steps in helping to prevent long-term complications. In addition, point out that physicians can now identify signs of physical complications much earlier, and that earlier detection and treatment may stop some complications from getting worse.

Discuss the many medical advances made over the past decades. Mention, for example, new oral medications, new types of insulin and schedules for insulin delivery, and new methods for monitoring blood glucose control, such as home blood glucose meters and the glycosylated hemoglobin test. When stable blood glucose control is maintained within the context of frequent medical follow-up, all of these new tools help to increase the patient's probability for a long and healthy life with diabetes. This may be a more optimistic message than many family members have heard before, and, therefore, it may need to be repeated and reinforced.

A second frequent fear of family members (that is much less discussed) is fear of low blood glucose. Seeing a loved one become incoherent or disoriented or have a seizure because of a low blood glucose reaction can be a terrifying experience for family members. Acknowledge this reality. Help family members understand that hypoglycemia is expected to occur in patients who are trying to improve their blood glucose control or are striving for tight control. Tell spouses that patients cannot always detect the warning signs of hypoglycemia, but that some patients can learn to detect their early warning signs more accurately (see Chapters 9 and 10). Point out to family members that placing blame or indicating disappointment when the patient has a low blood glucose reaction only compounds the problem. Most importantly, teach family members to support the patient by readily stopping an activity so that the patient can check his or her blood glucose level or have a snack.

Family members need to understand what hypoglycemia feels like to the patient, and they need to realize that the patient may behave differently when experiencing it. Low blood glucose levels may cause moodiness or negative behavior in the patient, or may make it unsafe, at times, for the patient to perform certain daily activities, such as driving, operating machinery, or caring for young children. Living with hypoglycemia and the threat of hypoglycemia are profound stresses on the family. Help families by anticipating and responding directly and realistically to the stress of hypoglycemia.

Family members can help patients in the prevention and treatment of hypoglycemia. Many family members feel helpless in the face of hypoglycemia. Therefore, it is important to tell them that by helping the patient prevent low blood glucose reactions, they are providing the most direct assistance possible. In some families, one person tries to see that the patient carries some fast-acting treatment for low blood glucose. Sometimes, a family member may carry a backup supply rather than ask or remind the patient. Some patients are helped when a family member reminds them to check their blood glucose. In other families, members learn to give glucagon just in case the patient has a severe low blood glucose reaction. Ask the patient and the family to decide what behaviors would work best for them.

To summarize this guideline about listening to the broad range of normal feelings—from fears of hypoglycemia to guilt over the diagnosis—that diabetes brings to all families, remember that while it is not necessary to supply answers for all of the family members' concerns, it is necessary and most useful to have family members voice their concerns and begin to try to solve some of these concerns.

Teach the Family What Is Realistic to Expect About the Patient's Blood Glucose Levels and Behavior

Teach family members that perfect blood glucose levels and perfect behavior are not possible goals in diabetes management. Similarly, help family members understand that patients with diabetes cannot always control their blood glucose levels, even if they are following their medical regimen. Without this foundation, family members assume that high and low blood glucose levels are *always* due to the patient's lack of behavioral control (e.g., "no will power," "lazy," etc.). When a family expects perfect blood glucose levels or diabetes management behavior from the patient, the patient is set up for failure and will experience more criticism and negative feedback from the family.

Help family members identify their unrealistic expectations for the patient's self-care behavior or for blood glucose levels or weight loss. Help family members see how having realistic expectations helps create more positive feelings between the patient and family members.

Teach Positive Family Involvement That Prevents Destructive Family Involvement

Positive family involvement supports the patient's diabetes self-care. Destructive family involvement undermines the patient's attempts at healthy diabetes self-care. The process of learning to give support and help must be worked out for each family. Teach family members to ask the patient questions like, "Does it help you stay on your meal plan when I suggest that we go to the cafeteria instead of the snack bar for lunch?"

A "miscarried helping cycle" can occur when well-meaning efforts of family members leave the patient feeling that family members lack confidence in him or her. Miscarried helping is when well-intentioned support attempts fail because they are excessive, untimely, or inappropriate. Second-guessing or arguing with the patient about his or her management decisions only undermines the patient's self-confidence and desire to make healthy choices. Even when family members know what to do, their helping effort may create a context that undermines the very objective they set out to achieve. Spouses and parents, especially, will feel frustrated that they cannot force the patient to make healthy choices all of the time. It is important to help families recognize that diabetes management at home will create conditions where the patient's motivation for self-care may become sidelined by the power of another struggle: that of preserving individual autonomy in the face of unwanted helping.

If a family is always arguing about "what is allowed on the meal plan," first ask the patient to define what family members could do to help him or her stay on the meal plan. It may be that not eating treats in front of the patient would help most, or that not eating all of the sugar-free ice cream out of the freezer would be a way family members could help. Helping may involve reminding or protecting the patient's special foods. Helping will be different with every patient and in every family. In miscarried helping, the original diabetes-related problem, such as the patient's need to adhere to a special meal plan, becomes lost or reframed. The helping process deteriorates when family members rely on strategies such as name-calling, insults, and other self-defeating behaviors. The patient feels shamed and blamed and increases his or her resistance. Everyone in the family has lost sight of the initial diabetes-related goal—the benefits to the patient of staying on a meal plan balanced with the medication.

In summary, it is not sufficient to simply tell family members they need to be helpful and supportive. Help define specific roles for each family member.

CONCLUSION

Family relationships play a vital, complex role in the lives of people with diabetes, and family support can have a positive effect on the metabolic control of the person with diabetes. For the clinician to begin to successfully involve family members in diabetes treatment, four principles are recommended:

1. Teach the family about diabetes in general.
2. Listen to the family's concerns, worries, and past experiences with diabetes.
3. Educate the family to have realistic and appropriate expectations concerning blood glucose levels and behavior.
4. Model positive helping and prevent destructive family helping that undermines the patient's attempts at healthy diabetes self-care.

Providing support is often a delicate and highly individualized process for each patient and his or her family. The needs of both the patient and the family members must be addressed and balanced. Clinicians can assist families in negotiating this complex process by talking openly about the roles of family members.

ACKNOWLEDGMENTS

Preparation of this manuscript was supported by the National Institute of Diabetes, Digestive, and Kidney Diseases Grant DK-R01-46887, by the Charles Hood Foundation, and by the Herbert Graetz Fund.

BIBLIOGRAPHY

Anderson BJ: Diabetes and adaptations in family systems. In *Neuropsychological and Behavioral Aspects of Insulin- and Non-Insulin-Dependent Diabetes.* Holmes CS, Ed. New York, Springer Verlag, 1990, p. 85–101

Anderson BJ: Working with families of patients on intensive insulin regimens. *Diabetes Spectrum* 8:69–70, 1995

Anderson BJ, Coyne JC: "Miscarried helping" in the families of children and adolescents with chronic diseases. In *Advances in Child Health Psychology.* Johnson J, Johnson S, Eds. Gainesville, University of Florida Press, 1991, p. 167–177

Baron RA: Negative effects of destructive criticism: impact on conflict, self-efficacy and task performance. *J Appl Psychol* 73:199–207, 1988

Polonsky WH: Besieged by the diabetes police. *Diabetes Self-Management* 12:21–26, 1995

Warram JH, Rich SS, Krolewski AS: Epidemiology and genetics of diabetes mellitus. In *Joslin's Diabetes Mellitus.* 13th ed. Kahn C, Weir G, Eds. Malvern, PA, Lea & Febiger, 1994, p. 210–215

TREATMENT REGIMEN FACTORS

As Glasgow and Eakins point out in their chapter, managing diabetes successfully can be one of life's most challenging tasks. These authors provide an overview of key self-management issues in an effort to help diabetes clinicians set priorities for change efforts and identify potentially effective intervention strategies. Glasgow and Eakins help us appreciate the wide range of factors that influence self-management behavior, and they offer practical recommendations for what can be accomplished during office visits.

Successfully managing the dietary demands and restrictions of life with diabetes is almost certainly the most common obstacle to effective self-management. In their chapter, Schlundt, Pichert, Gregory, and Davis offer recommendations for an individualized, patient-centered approach to dietary management that integrates ethnic and cultural as well as individual considerations. This approach is based on the guidelines recently published by the American Diabetes Association for the nutritional management of diabetes. The authors provide a comprehensive guide to assessing lifestyle and diet and to effective behavioral interventions in this critical area of self-care.

Exercise is another area of self-management that is problematic for many people with diabetes. Marrero and

Sizemore discuss the benefits of consistent regular exercise for people with either type I or type II diabetes. They also offer specific guidelines for helping patients select the right exercise program and for helping patients maintain their motivation to exercise. In addition, the authors provide information on risks and recommendations for exercising with diabetes complications.

The Diabetes Control and Complications Trial (DCCT) established unequivocally the benefits of lowering blood glucose to near-normal levels for people with type I diabetes, but it also documented the increased risk of severe hypoglycemia associated with intensive treatment. In their chapters, Cox, Gonder-Frederick, and Clarke provide us with information and techniques to help patients cope more effectively with hypoglycemia. Their research group has studied hypoglycemia in people with type I diabetes since 1980. Based on their research, the authors developed an intervention called blood glucose awareness training (BGAT), which has been shown to increase an individual's ability to recognize, avoid, and treat hypoglycemia. The first of the two chapters on hypoglycemia addresses the problem of low blood glucose and its psychosocial consequences, as well as hypoglycemic symptoms and hypoglycemic unawareness. The second chapter focuses on issues of prevention and treatment.

Dealing With Diabetes Self-Management

6

Russell E. Glasgow, PhD, and
Elizabeth G. Eakin, PhD

INTRODUCTION

Managing diabetes successfully can be one of life's most challenging tasks. It is the rare individual who manages key lifestyle tasks, such as healthy eating or regular physical activity, well. Even more challenging is combining these tasks with the multitude of other tasks of the diabetes regimen. New data on the staggering health-care costs associated with diabetes complications and evidence from the Diabetes Control and Complications Trial (DCCT) and other trials show that tight control and diabetes self-management can reduce many of these costly complications. Such findings make it imperative that patients are helped to self-manage their disease. All too often, however, the difficulty of coping with the demands of the diabetes regimen can overwhelm both patients and clinicians. This chapter provides a framework and practical suggestions for facilitating diabetes self-management.

SELF-MANAGEMENT INFLUENCES, TASKS, AND CONSEQUENCES

Figure 1 is intended to help providers better understand key self-management issues, set priorities for change efforts, and identify intervention strategies. Factors influencing diabetes self-management are

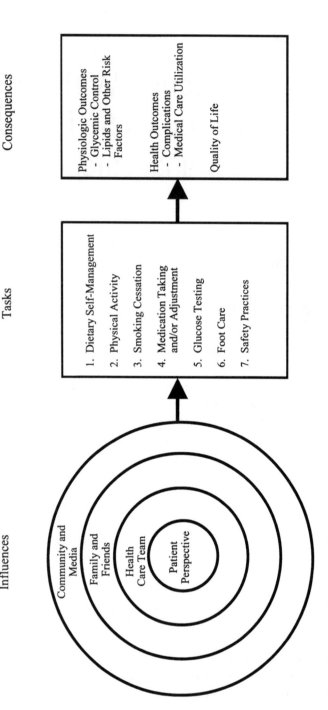

FIGURE 1. Diabetes self-management influences, tasks, and consequences.

shown on the left side of the figure. These factors are arranged in concentric circles based upon their proximity to the patient. These different levels of influence will be discussed, in turn, in terms of what to assess and what can be done for intervention. For now it is sufficient to note that there are multiple levels of influence that combine to determine self-management. And by implication, effective self-management is *not* achieved simply by providing patients with knowledge, but rather by addressing motivations, beliefs, coping skills, and environmental support as well.

The center of the figure represents several different tasks of the diabetes regimen. These tasks are represented separately to illustrate that there is usually little relationship between the extent to which a patient follows one aspect of the regimen and his or her level of self-care in other areas. Stated differently: there are few uniformly "good or bad compliers." Most patients show variability in the extent to which they follow different regimen recommendations. It is important to assess the degree of self-management in each area (and not to overwhelm the patient with trying to change everything at once).

Finally, the consequences of self-management, including glycemic control, health outcomes, quality of life, and medical care utilization are shown on the right side of the figure. Self-management and diabetes control are not the same: self-management is one of the multiple determinants of health outcomes (along with genetics, regimen prescriptions, and other factors). One cannot judge a patient's level of self-care from his or her HbA_{1c} level.

The main point of Figure 1 is the importance of personalizing the aspect(s) of self-management one needs to target and determining which sets of influences are most relevant or possible to change at a given time. The figure also helps one to appreciate the complexity and difficulty of diabetes self-management and demonstrates the inappropriateness of dichotomizing patients into "good and bad compliers."

ASSESSMENT AND INTERVENTION STRATEGIES

Although there are times when a comprehensive approach to self-management is optimal (e.g., upon initial diagnosis, when initiating intensive therapy with a multidisciplinary team), at most visits, clinicians have neither the time nor the resources to focus on several

TABLE 1. *Self-Management Assessment and Intervention Guidelines*

Patient Factors

♦ Assess the patient's belief that diabetes is serious and that what he or she does to manage it makes a difference.

♦ Provide personalized feedback on specific effects of diabetes on the patient's health (e.g., "Did you know that diabetes is one of the major risk factors for developing heart disease?").

♦ Educate the patient on the potential benefits of specific self-management behaviors (e.g., "Regular physical activity helps diabetes control by . . .").

Health-Care Team Issues

♦ Reinforce the same patient goal(s) at a given visit.

♦ Note in the patient's chart the self-management issues to be followed up on at the next contact.

♦ Provide follow-up support via phone calls and reviewing goals at subsequent visits.

Social Environment

♦ Assess the patient's barriers to self-management goals (e.g., "Ms. Jones, what things might interfere with you following the blood glucose testing plan we developed today?").

♦ Help the patient enlist resources available to deal with barriers identified (e.g., "Are you aware of the diabetes support group at the hospital? I think that you might find it quite helpful to be able to talk to others who are dealing with many of the same issues.").

---

different targets. Also, patients will have greater success if they focus on one or two behaviors between visits.

Table 1 and the discussion below provide practical recommendations for what can be accomplished *during office visits* related to each level of influence on diabetes self-management pictured in Figure 1.

Patient Factors

The most important factors in determining self-management goals are the patient's perspective on the diabetes regimen and what changes he or she considers reasonable and realistic. Two important beliefs to listen for are that patients: 1) consider their diabetes to be serious and 2) believe that what they do makes a difference. Common experiences in living with diabetes, such as health behaviors of family members and friends, work and social schedules and pressures, and implicit and explicit messages from one's health-care team and the media, can either promote or interfere with establishment of such beliefs. Patients who don't hold these beliefs will likely not be motivated to engage in diabetes self-management behaviors. Such patients may need additional personalized feedback on the specific implications of diabetes for their health. They may also need education on the potential benefits of specific self-management behaviors.

In particular, it is important to see if patients consider lifestyle aspects of diabetes management (e.g., diet and exercise) as important as medical aspects (e.g., taking medication and testing glucose). If they do not, they will be unlikely to follow through with the challenges of lifestyle modification. For example, we have heard patients exclaim, "I knew that smoking was bad in general, but I assumed that if it was important for *me* to quit, my doctor would have told me."

Health-Care Team Issues

The core issue here is consistency and reinforcement of patient goals across different health-care team members. Rather than having the physician emphasize medication, the nurse stress glucose testing, and the dietitian recommend major dietary changes, success is more likely if all team members reinforce a common goal, such as foot care, for that visit.

The patient needs to leave a given visit with a clear idea (and, if possible, a written "contract sheet") of the key goal(s) for the next visit. When patients are given assignments, it is particularly important to review and comment on any records that have been kept at the next visit or contact.

The Social Environment

It is important to assess and incorporate into treatment the patients' anticipated barriers to self-management goals and available resources. This can be accomplished either by asking the patient what he or she thinks might interfere with the self-management goal for the next visit (e.g., "Ms. Smith, what things do you think might make it difficult for you to follow the eating plan we discussed today?") or by having the patient complete a brief "barriers checklist." The clinician can then help the patient develop possible solutions, focusing on the use of available family, friend, and community resources.

Most communities offer free or low-cost support or reinforcement activities (e.g., ADA meetings, hospital or HMO lectures or education programs, newsletters) that can extend the motivation patients receive during office visits. Other community support options to reinforce provider messages about diabetes management include activity programs (e.g., mall walking) and diabetes and other chronic disease support groups (in person or via the Internet).

Self-management activities do not occur in a vacuum, but rather in a social context. If maintenance of self-management is to be expected, follow-up support must be arranged in the form of family and community social support and follow-up contacts with members of the healthcare team. Recent research demonstrates the cost-effectiveness of follow-up telephone calls from staff in improving maintenance of behavior change.

AN EXAMPLE OF A BRIEF OFFICE-BASED SELF-MANAGEMENT PROGRAM

Our research team is currently completing an evaluation of a dietary self-management program being conducted during regular office visits. Through the use of focused assessment instruments and modern computer technology, we conduct a highly personalized intervention that addresses each of the self-management issues discussed above. This intervention requires only 20 minutes of additional time from the patient (and nurse or dietitian) and no additional time from the physician. The following description relies on relatively sophisticated touch-screen computer technology (which we feel will become commonplace in most medical offices over the next several years). However, these same issues can be addressed almost as efficiently face to face or by telephone or mail contacts.

Table 2 summarizes the key self-management issues to be addressed irrespective of the intervention and assessment medium (face to face, computer, telephone, or mail).

Through the use of touch-screen computerized assessment, we identify specific dietary self-management behaviors leading to high saturated fat intake. The patient perspective is addressed through assessment of patient beliefs about the seriousness of diabetes and

T A B L E 2 . *Key Self-Management Issues to Address During Office Visits*

1. Identify specific self-management targets.
♦ Assess self-management behaviors and glycemic control separately because they are different things.
♦ Assess adherence to different aspects of the diabetes regimen.

2. Elicit and listen to the patient's perspective.
♦ Ask which things the patient is ready to work on.
♦ Assess the patient's beliefs about diabetes severity and helpfulness of various regimen activities.

3. Work as a team.
♦ Provide feedback on assessment results to the patient and other team members.
♦ Reinforce the importance of a consistent goal, rather than having the patient try to do many things at one visit.

4. Arrange social support for diabetes self-management.
♦ Plan for how to deal with barriers to self-care.
♦ Enlist the support of family, friends, and/or local organizations.
♦ Provide follow-up phone calls or other communications between visits (e.g., fax, modem transmissions).

about the importance of dietary management. Patients are allowed a choice of areas to address and goals to work toward as well. Social-environmental influences (e.g., family members eating foods not on the patient's diet in front of the patient) are addressed by touch-screen assessment of perceived barriers to low-fat eating.

Patient/health-care team interactions are facilitated by a one-page computer-generated feedback form that summarizes key self-management issues for the patient (Table 3) and by a separate one-page computer printout that summarizes patient self-management behaviors, beliefs about diabetes control, recommended goal areas, and laboratory results for the provider (Table 4). The physician is asked to provide only a two-sentence message about the importance of dietary self-management and a recommendation to meet with another clinician to develop a personalized plan immediately following the physician exam.

The 20-minute self-management session focuses on the use of the above assessment information to negotiate a personalized behavioral goal with patients, collaboratively plan strategies to overcome likely barriers to this goal, and mutually develop a goal-setting contract. To

TABLE 3. *Overcoming Barriers to Healthy Eating (Patient Feedback)*

For: Joe

Personalized Dietary Goal for the Next Few Months: To avoid fat as a flavoring or seasoning.

Type of Situation That Is Most Challenging: Social/Schedule.
Specific situations:
1. Eating at a restaurant that has few appropriate choices.
2. Social event where there is a lot of food not on your eating plan.

Other Situations That Make It Difficult for You to Follow Your Diet:
1. The recommended healthy foods cause you digestive problems.
2. Feeling a strong craving for a certain high-fat food.

How You Might Prepare for Problem Situations (From Discussion With Your Health-Care Team):
1. _____
2. _____
3. _____

Benefits of Good Diabetes Self-Management to Remind Yourself About (Complete and Refer to Often):
1. _____
2. _____
3. _____

---

bridge the time until the next quarterly office visit, two brief follow-up phone calls are made to reinforce patients' progress and help solve any difficulties.

CONCLUSION

The intervention described above makes substantial use of video and computer technology. Even more sophisticated and efficient technology will likely be available in the near future with the advent of computerized medical records, automatic provider prompts, pen-based computing, etc. The primary point is not the technology involved— paper-and-pencil versions of the instruments could be completed by

TABLE 4. *Mckenzie Health/Oregon Research Institute Personalized Diabetes Assessment Summary Form (Provider Feedback)*

Patient Name: Joe	**ID#:** 547		**Date:** 3/6/96

Issue Patient Would Most Like to Discuss This Visit:

_____

_____

		Level	**Date**
Weight: 198	**Height:** 5'9"		
Percent of Ideal Weight: 134	**Blood Pressure:**		
Smoking Status: Smoker	**Cholesterol:**	234	3/6/96
Exercise Status: Active	**HbA$_{1c}$:**		

Primary Nutrition Goal for the Next Few Months: To avoid fat as a flavoring or seasoning.

Key Obstacles Patient Has for Managing Diet:

_____

_____

♦ **Key Message for Patient:** Following a healthy low-fat eating pattern is one of the most important things you can do for your health.

the patient in the waiting room—but, rather, that a highly personalized intervention can be conducted in a brief period of time.

Key features of the medical office-based intervention are that it 1) addresses the multiple levels of influence on diabetes self-management shown in Figure 1 and 2) incorporates many of the recommended practices in Table 1. Probably the single most important thing is that a realistic goal is generated by and makes sense to the patient and is repeatedly reinforced by all members of the health-care team.

ACKNOWLEDGMENTS

Preparation of this manuscript was supported by Grant 3DK-R01-35524 from the National Institutes of Diabetes, Digestive, and Kidney Diseases.

BIBLIOGRAPHY

Anderson LA, Jenkins CM (Eds.): Educational innovations in diabetes: Where are we now? *Diabetes Spectrum* 7:90–124, 1994

Anderson RM, Funnell MM: The role of the physician in patient education. *Pract Diabetol* May/June:10–12, 1990

Bradley C: *Handbook of Psychology and Diabetes: A Guide to Psychological Measurement in Diabetes Research and Practice.* Chur, Switzerland, Harwood Academic Publishers, 1994

Clement S: Diabetes self-management education. *Diabetes Care* 18: 1204–1214, 1995

Glasgow RE: A practical model of diabetes management and education. *Diabetes Care* 18:117–126, 1995

Glasgow RE, Toobert DJ, Hampson SE, Noell JW: A brief office-based intervention to facilitate diabetes dietary self-management. *Health Educ Res*, 1995

Litzelman DK, Slemenda CW, Langefeld CD, Hays LM, Welch MA, Bild DE, Ford ES, Vinicor F: Reduction of lower extremity clinical abnormalities in patients with non-insulin-dependent diabetes mellitus: a randomized, controlled trial. *Ann Intern Med* 119:36–41, 1993

Raymond M: *The Human Side of Diabetes: Beyond Doctors, Diets, and Drugs.* Chicago, Noble Press, 1992

Rubin RR, Biermann J, Toohey B: *Psyching Out Diabetes: A Positive Approach to Your Negative Emotions.* Los Angeles, RGA Publishing Group, 1992

Eating and Diabetes: A Patient-Centered Approach

7

David G. Schlundt, PhD, James W. Pichert, PhD, Becky Gregory, RD, and Dianne Davis, RD

INTRODUCTION

In people with diabetes, moment-to-moment blood glucose fluctuates, sometimes dramatically, with insulin action, physical activity, and food intake. Of these three influences, food intake is often the most challenging and difficult to manage for patients and clinicians alike. Historically, routine medical management included prescribing structured diets and telling patients to follow them. This simplistic approach has frustrated both health-care providers, who complain that most patients do not adhere, and people with diabetes, who complain that traditional diet prescriptions are unrealistic and impossible to follow long term. Fortunately, alternatives to simplistic, structured diets are proving possible, feasible, and desirable. This chapter describes a workable patient-centered approach to diabetes nutritional management now advocated by most diabetes experts.

WHAT IS PATIENT-CENTERED DIABETES CARE?

The goals of nutrition therapy in diabetes are to

- Maintain near-normal blood glucose levels.
- Achieve optimum serum lipid levels.

- Provide adequate calories for growth and/or maintenance of a reasonable body weight.
- Prevent acute and chronic complications of diabetes.
- Promote wellness through optimal nutrition.

To better meet these goals, the American Diabetes Association recently published a new set of nutrition guidelines for the management of diabetes. The guidelines call for an individualized, patient-centered approach that integrates nutrition therapy into the patient's lifestyle with sensitivity to ethnic, cultural, and individual differences.

Instead of the traditional approach of prescribing specific numbers or percentages of calories, carbohydrates, protein, and fats, patient-centered nutrition management involves

- Assessing the patient's current eating habits, insulin or medication use, and patterns of exercise and physical activity.
- Starting with current lifestyle and negotiating a medical management plan that will achieve good control with an acceptable degree of lifestyle change.
- Sharing realistic expectations concerning the difficulty of meeting glucose targets in everyday situations.
- Sustaining lifelong self-management practices that minimize complications while maximizing quality of life.
- Teaching behavioral strategies that help patients achieve and sustain successes in daily life.

ASSESSING EATING PATTERNS AND LIFESTYLE

Before a plan can be negotiated, the provider must understand the patient's current eating habits: the what, when, where, why, and how much each patient eats. Foods do not just fill our stomachs, and they are much more than blends of micronutrients and macronutrients. Foods have cultural, interpersonal, and emotional meanings. Understanding the various meanings foods have for an individual and how life circumstances influence food choices will help in negotiating a realistic plan of diabetes self-management.

Table 1 presents common lifestyle influences on dietary adherence. Each entry represents a type of everyday situation that makes adher-

TABLE 1. *Assessing Lifestyle and Diet*

Type of Problem	Description	Interview Questions
Negative Emotions	The patient overeats to cope with stress and negative feelings.	Are there any situations in your life that are currently causing you a lot of stress? Do you eat differently when you feel upset, depressed, or stressed?
Resisting Temptation	Foods, cues, and cravings are tempting the patient to eat inappropriate foods.	What foods or situations trigger cravings? What foods or situations tempt you to eat inappropriately?
Eating Out	Eating away from home (e.g., restaurants) makes it hard for the patient to control what and how much he or she eats.	How do the amounts or kinds of foods you eat differ when you eat away from home or at a restaurant?
Feeling Deprived	The patient feels he or she cannot eat certain foods he or she enjoys and is tempted to give up and give in.	How often do you feel like giving up on taking good care of your diabetes because it keeps you from eating the way you enjoy? What foods do you feel like you should give up eating?
Time Pressure	Having many demands on the patient's time makes healthy eating difficult.	What kinds of social, family, or job pressures make it hard for you to find the time to eat the way you want to?
Tempted to Relapse	The patient feels discouraged or feels like a failure and considers no longer trying to eat right.	How often do you feel so discouraged about your eating plan that you want to just give up? Do you see your current plan as rigid or flexible?
Planning	A hectic schedule makes it hard for the patient to plan what and when to eat.	How difficult is it for you to plan when, where, and what you will eat?
Competing Priorities	Many responsibilities and obligations (e.g., family and job) interfere with the patient's ability to make healthy food choices.	What important priorities in your life get in the way of making healthy food choices? Do you sometimes feel like you have to choose between good diabetes care and other important life goals?
Social Events	The patient overeats at parties, holidays, special occasions, and other social events that involve food.	How do the amounts or kinds of foods you eat differ when you eat at parties or social events?
Family Support	The patient's family does not support healthy food choices.	Describe the things your family does to support or hinder your efforts to eat the way you want to.
Food Refusal	Someone offers an inappropriate food and the patient finds it hard to refuse.	How hard is it for you to refuse food when someone offers it to you?
Friend's Support	The patient's friends do not support healthy food choices.	Describe the things your friends do to support or hinder your efforts to eat the way you want to.

Adapted from Schlundt DG, Rea MR, Kline SS, Pichert JW: Situational obstacles to dietary adherence for adults with diabetes. *J Am Diet Assoc* 94:874–876, 1994.

ence difficult, and each entry suggests interview questions to use during an assessment.

BUILDING MEDICAL MANAGEMENT AROUND LIFESTYLE

Patient-centered nutrition and medical management in diabetes involves the following key elements:

Glucose monitoring and target ranges. Managing blood glucose requires

1. Frequent feedback on current serum glucose level
2. An agreeable schedule for self-monitoring of blood glucose
3. Negotiated blood glucose target ranges: target ranges depend on the patient's degree of control desired, risk for hypoglycemia, commitment to preventing complications, and resources and abilities
4. Access to monitoring equipment and supplies
5. Training in the appropriate use of equipment

Quantifying food intake. To regulate blood glucose, patients need to learn to use a method for quantifying their food intake. Commonly used strategies include exchange groups, carbohydrate gram counting, and total available glucose (TAG). Patients with type II diabetes who want to lose weight may also benefit from learning to count fat grams and/or calories. Choose a strategy that reflects the patient's goals, abilities, and preferences. Any of these methods can be used to help patients make intelligent food choices and diabetes management decisions.

Making adjustments in food, insulin, and activity. When a person has a very stable and routine lifestyle, it may be possible to take the same insulin, eat the same amount of food, and engage in consistent physical activity such that adjustments rarely need to be made to keep blood glucose in the target range. Most patients, however, will need to learn how to adjust food, activity, and/or insulin to compensate for blood glucose levels outside the target range. All patients taking insulin must know how to use glucose or appropriate foods to quickly and effectively treat hypoglycemia.

Problem-solving: the ongoing process of monitoring and adjusting. Table 1 identifies many everyday situations in which decisions have to be made and actions implemented to keep blood glucose in the target range. Patient-centered diabetes management includes helping people learn how to anticipate, prevent, and solve daily problems as they arise. The process is one of frequent self-monitoring of blood glucose and adjusting of food, insulin, or activity to cope with each situation.

Patient choice and flexibility in goals. No single approach to nutrition management will work for everyone. For diabetes care to be effective, patients must participate in selecting their goals and strategies. Some patients will prefer relatively structured approaches with a fixed insulin dose and a well-defined meal plan. Other patients will prefer the flexibility of adjusting insulin to match carbohydrate consumption. In a patient-centered approach, the range of options is discussed and a plan is tailored to the individual's needs and preferences.

In general, the same self-management principles for people on insulin apply to type II diabetes patients who are not using insulin. Besides strategies for keeping blood glucose in a target range, the management of type II diabetes may include efforts to lose weight, reduce fat intake, optimally space meal times, and/or increase exercise. Losing weight and improving fitness require individually negotiated goals, flexibility in how to achieve these goals, and ability to solve problems using self-monitoring and adjustment. Long-term maintenance of a healthy weight is the most difficult problem in the nutrition management of type II diabetes. Individualized goals, flexibility, and ongoing problem-solving are critical for lasting success.

Be realistic. Patient-centered diabetes management requires realistic expectations.

Expect compromise. Even starting with a person's current lifestyle, it is unrealistic to think no changes will have to be made. People whose lifestyles are erratic, haphazard, high stress, or in some way incompatible with even the most flexible of diabetes management plans will have to compromise. Both patient and provider, however, will compromise as they negotiate a workable self-management plan.

Skills are learned gradually. Diabetes self-management requires many skills, such as self-monitoring of blood glucose, use of a sliding insulin scale, counting carbohydrate grams, being more assertive with family members, and so forth. Expect people to need time to master these skills. While learning, people need feedback, encouragement, and patience.

Slips and relapses are common. Changes in lifestyle do not automatically become permanent. It is common for patients to fall short of their goals from time to time. Long-term success involves monitoring, adjusting, and problem-solving in ever-changing circumstances that challenge an individual's ability to keep blood glucose in the target range. Teach patients to expect difficulty, to plan ahead for it, and to seek support when trouble occurs. Perfect performance in all situations is unrealistic.

Problems will not go away if you ignore them. Difficulties, relapses, and stressful episodes occur in everyone's life. Ignoring these problems will not make them go away. Many patients, however, use the strategy of denial when faced with difficulties. Sometimes, the first task is to help a patient admit that there is a problem.

The key to realistic expectations is reasonable goals. Frequent contact and fostering honest and open communication facilitate long-term success. Accept problems when they occur and work to solve them. Avoid blaming, scolding, and scaring people. These negative strategies rarely work, if ever. Ask instead, "What are you willing and able to do to get your blood glucose under better control?" (See Chapter 17 for more on patient-centered care and the empowerment approach.)

DIETARY SELF-MANAGEMENT

Diet instruction should 1) facilitate good diabetes control and 2) foster wellness through healthy eating habits. Advances in self-monitoring of blood glucose, types of insulin, and insulin delivery regimens make it unnecessary for people to be forced to follow a rigid diet. Instead of emphasizing diets, focus on appropriate self-management. Ultimately, each person is responsible for what he or she eats and drinks and for the health outcomes resulting from these choices. Self-management means a person learns to modify choices in order to meet short-term and long-term health goals.

The primary concern for patients with diabetes is achieving adequate blood glucose control. However, patients with diabetes are at higher risk for heart disease than the general population. Dietary self-management, therefore, may also mean learning to make food and beverage choices that lower the risk of heart disease. Success in reducing heart disease risk involves knowledge, motivation, skill, and persistence. One must know what foods to emphasize and which to limit. Since many other goals and priorities compete with healthy eating for a person's time and attention, a strong commitment to healthy eating is required. Skills like reading food labels, counting fat grams, ordering a low-fat meal in a restaurant, modifying recipes, or overcoming long-standing problems with binge eating may have to be mastered. Prevention of heart disease is a lifelong process, and persistence is necessary to overcome a constant stream of situations that challenge one's knowledge, skill, and commitment to healthy eating.

Flexibility, realistic goals, and ongoing support are more important than factual education in helping people master dietary self-management. Each person is different, each faces unique challenges, and each proceeds at his or her own pace toward the long-term goals of good diabetes care.

DIETARY RULES OF THUMB

Consider teaching patients the following five behavioral guidelines for successful dietary self-management:

1. **Be consistent.** The more predictable the timing, composition, and size of meals, the less decision-making and adjustment required. Consistent habits are the basis of a successful plan for diabetes care.

2. **When you can't be consistent, be close.** When eating the usual amounts or kinds of foods is impossible, choosing similar foods makes for less adjustment and decision-making.
3. **When you aren't close, make adjustments.** Often, circumstances lead to deviations in the amount, composition, or timing of meals. On these occasions, problem-solving and decision-making are needed to identify and implement adjustments that will quickly return blood glucose to the target range.
4. **Be prepared, plan ahead.** Many difficulties can be avoided by looking ahead and making plans to be prepared.
5. **Avoid all-or-none thinking.** When deviations, unexpected difficulties, or circumstances requiring problem-solving and adjustment arise, do not look on these times as instances of failure. Replace the kind of black-and-white thinking that sees choices as either successes or failures with realistic goals, self-acceptance, and moderation.

There is no one best way to solve self-management problems. In practice, people must be flexible and make compromises, approaching problems with a hierarchy of strategies ranging from choosing consistent meals to making complex regimen adjustments.

ROLE OF THE DIABETES TEAM

Teaching dietary self-management involves assessment, negotiating goals, identifying skill deficits, providing education and skill training, along with ongoing support and follow-up. Developing problem-solving skills is also important for the health professional. Obviously, these goals are impossible to accomplish in a 15-minute doctor's visit. Success involves a team approach. Patient-centered diabetes care requires

1. A well-trained team of qualified professionals.
2. A case manager for each patient who is responsible for ensuring that the expertise of the other team members is used as needed.
3. Open lines of communication between the patient and the team, and among team members.
4. A commitment to basing decisions on what will be best for the patient rather than what will be most convenient for the providers.

Implementing patient-centered diabetes care is not easy. Just as patients face many obstacles in achieving good glycemic control, treatment teams will face many obstacles in implementing patient-centered team management, such as third-party reimbursement, distinctions between disciplinary domains of expertise, institutional pressures to see more patients in less time, cultural and economic barriers that separate patient from professional, and the effects of professional stress and burnout.

CONCLUSION

Simplistic diabetes nutritional management involves handing patients a "canned" diet and urging strict adherence. That approach requires little time or imagination from the health-care professional, but it almost always frustrates and fails the patient. A patient-centered approach, involving individualized assessment, goal negotiation, and problem-solving, is far more time-consuming and intellectually challenging for both patients and health professionals, but its chances for success are much higher. Patients who can routinely adjust their food, activity, and/or insulin to life's ever-changing circumstances will achieve better blood glucose control and will suffer less resentment. In addition, patients and clinicians will enjoy better relationships: many patients will come to see their health-care team as an advocate and ally in their diabetes management. We hope clinicians will adopt this perspective on diabetes nutrition management and adapt our suggestions to their patients.

ACKNOWLEDGMENTS

This work was supported by National Institutes of Health Grant P60-DK-20593.

BIBLIOGRAPHY

American Diabetes Association: Nutrition recommendations and principles for people with diabetes mellitus. *Diabetes Care* (Suppl. 1) 19:S16–S19, 1996

The DCCT Research Group: Nutrition interventions for intensive therapy in the Diabetes Control and Complications Trial. *J Am Diet Assoc* 93:768–772, 1993

Gregory RP, Davis DL: Use of carbohydrate counting for meal planning in type I diabetes. *The Diabetes Educator* 20:406–409, 1994

Schlundt DG, Rea MR, Kline SS, Pichert JW: Situational obstacles to dietary adherence for adults with diabetes. *J Am Diet Assoc* 94:874–876, 1994

Tinker LF, Heins JM, Holler HJ: Commentary and translation: 1994 nutrition recommendations for diabetes. *J Am Diet Assoc* 94:507–511, 1994

Motivating Patients With Diabetes to Exercise

8

David G. Marrero, PhD, and
Jill M. Sizemore, MS

> *Exercise in the days before insulin we regarded as useful, but by no means did we appreciate it as vital in the care of diabetes....We should return to it to help us in the treatment of all of our cases....*
>
> (Joslin et al., *Treatment of Diabetes Mellitus, 1959*)

INTRODUCTION

Increasing evidence supports what Joslin observed nearly 40 years ago: a consistent, regular exercise program has many benefits for people with both type I and type II diabetes. Exercise has been shown to help people with diabetes lose weight, reduce their need for insulin and/or oral hypoglycemic agents, and improve glycemic control, thereby reducing the risk of complications. However, in spite of these benefits, many patients with diabetes do not use regular exercise as an integral part of their therapy.

Health-care professionals are in a unique and influential position to help inactive patients find the motivation to begin and maintain an effective and safe long-term exercise program. In this chapter, we offer suggestions as to how best to accomplish this goal. These suggestions are based on three intuitively simple, yet often neglected, axioms:

1. Promote a program that is intrinsically desirable and reinforcing for patients.

2. Recommend a program that is realistic, feasible, and sustainable for patients.
3. Educate patients on how to avoid the potential negative consequences of exercise, particularly those associated specifically with diabetes.

PROMOTING A PROGRAM THAT IS DESIRABLE AND REINFORCING

To understand how to motivate patients to exercise, consider these three basic principles of behavior modification that shape their decision to do so.

1. **Perceived benefits.** The first and most basic principle is that motivation to begin any new behavior, such as a regular exercise program, is grounded in one's perception of the benefits of that behavior and the importance of obtaining those benefits. An important corollary of this principle is that what one perceives as a benefit is idiosyncratic and can change over time.
2. **Perceived costs.** The second principle is that a behavior is not likely to be initiated or maintained if the costs associated with the activity outweigh the benefits. Furthermore, costs are idiosyncratically defined and can include physical, social, or psychological factors.
3. **Reinforcement.** The third principle is that if a behavior, such as exercising, leads to desired benefits, the behavior is reinforced in value and more likely to be repeated. If, on the other hand, the behavior does not lead to desired benefits or is seen as punishing, the behavior diminishes in value and, thus, is not likely to be repeated.

   A corollary of this principle is that reinforcement and punishment are most effective when they are applied immediately following the target behavior. The greater the delay, the weaker the motivating aspects. A second corollary is that in almost all cases, positive reinforcement paradigms are more effective in encouraging long-term behavior change than is the use of punishments.

Many patients do not have realistic expectations of the benefits and costs associated with exercise and may not understand how physical activity can help to reduce complication risk. Others attempt to exercise but experience physical discomfort, hypoglycemia, or injury, thus learning that the short-term costs outweigh the potential, long-term benefits.

Many health-care providers also fail to capitalize on the inherently motivating power of obtaining positive reinforcement when discussing exercise with patients. Frequently, the rationale for exercise is as a means to avoid complications, not as an intrinsically enjoyable activity that has health benefits. The motivating power of this rationale is further diminished in that the threatened punishment often won't occur for several years.

BUILDING THE FOUNDATION FOR MOTIVATION

To begin the process of motivating patients, recommend a regular exercise program and explain that the recommendation is based on extensive research that demonstrates several benefits of exercise for people in general and for people with diabetes in particular. These benefits include:

1. Health benefits, such as improvements in glucose regulation, weight control, lipid profiles, hypertension, and increased work capacity.
2. Social benefits, such as increased interaction with family members, "social others" (i.e., training partners), and participation in organized, community-based activities.
3. Psychological benefits, most notably anxiety, depression, stress reduction, and increased feelings of well-being.

However, to maximize the probability of motivating patients to begin an exercise program, it is important to also emphasize these several key points:

- Exercise is part of a lifelong management program. Tell patients not to expect to begin exercising at a high intensity. Help them select a series of goals that are safe and achievable, and that will help them to develop an effective program over time.
- Teach patients how to exercise properly, i.e., to perform the activity so that they avoid discomfort, injury, and problems with their diabetes. This will require that they be willing to experiment a bit with some new behaviors, including adjusting their diabetes regimen.

- Assure patients that they don't have to figure out how to do this alone. Health-care professionals are there to help them accomplish these goals.
- The key to patients sustaining an exercise program is in selecting one that is responsive to their personal situation: their goals, their desires, and the availability of time and appropriate support.

Having laid this foundation, clinicians will be ready to help patients select an exercise program that is likely to be a source of positive reinforcement and thus sustained over time.

HELPING PATIENTS SELECT THE RIGHT EXERCISE PROGRAM

Frequently, when patients are told to exercise by a clinician, it is a generic prescription with little or no guidance concerning what to do or how to do it. By discussing with patients their answers to two simple, related questions, clinicians can help them to more critically consider factors that can contribute to or inhibit their selection of an exercise method that they are likely to enjoy. These two questions are:

1. **What are your goals for exercise?** Finding out the patient's goals makes it easier to identify the types of activities that will help him or her achieve those goals. Whatever the goals, do not be judgmental. The patient's rationale might not reflect the clinician's personal feelings about what is most important for the patient, but may result in achieving the same end point.
2. **What types of physical activity do you like or think you would like to do?** This question is designed to help guide patients in selecting an appropriate activity that they are motivated to do. If they do not have a strong sense for what they want, a useful strategy is to ask them to indicate their preference between the following options:

   - Long- or short-duration exercise
   - High- versus low-intensity exercise
   - Exercising alone or with others
   - Exercising at home or at a facility
   - Exercising indoors versus outdoors
   - A competitive or cooperative sport

Try providing patients with a list of activities to stimulate their consideration of possible modes of exercise. Once a patient has narrowed down the possibilities, or even selected a specific exercise method, help him or her address the second axiom: the exercise program must be realistic and feasible in order for it to be sustained. This may be done by encouraging patients to consider what we term the "Ease of Access" and "Ease of Performance" index. These are self-assessments of how realistic the activity is for a patient, given his or her lifestyle.

THE EASE OF ACCESS AND EASE OF PERFORMANCE INDEX

Ease of Access Index

The Ease of Access Index addresses the question, "How easily can I engage in my activity of choice where I live?" Many people have a tendency to begin an exercise program only to find that it's simply too difficult to participate in on a regular basis for a variety of reasons that were either ignored, rationalized, or simply not considered before the program was begun. To determine a patient's Ease of Access Index for a given activity, ask the patient to consider the following questions:

- Does it require special facilities, and are these facilities accessible?
- Does it require special equipment, and is this equipment available and affordable?
- Does it require special training or instruction, and is this instruction readily available, scheduled at convenient times, easy to get to, and affordable?
- Does it require others to do it, and will I always be able to find partners when I want or need to play?
- Is it seasonal, and what will I do other times of the year?

Ease of Performance Index

If the exercise activity of interest has an acceptable Ease of Access Index, encourage patients to evaluate it in terms of its Ease of Performance Index. The Ease of Performance Index considers the question, "How suitable is a specific activity given my physical attributes and lifestyle?" To determine the Ease of Performance Index, ask the patient to consider the following questions:

- Do I have physical limitations that make a given activity not suitable for me?
- Can I realistically integrate my chosen activity into my lifestyle?
- Can I realistically afford any costs associated with it?
- Do I have a good support network if I need one for my activity?

The first question is most critical for people with diabetes. Before patients begin any exercise, they need to be aware of physical limitations that may affect their ability to engage in the activity. Have all people with diabetes undergo a medical examination to determine whether there are any musculoskeletal/orthopedic concerns that may rule out various exercise activities. Similarly, identify any existing comorbidities and complications, such as neuropathy, retinopathy, nephropathy, and cardiovascular disease, and consider them in the exercise prescription.

In addition to the physical examination, a graded exercise test (either a step test, bicycle or arm ergometer test, treadmill test, or the stress EKG) to measure cardiorespiratory fitness before beginning an exercise program is also recommended for some individuals. The exercise test not only determines contraindications to exercise, but also greatly facilitates the exercise prescription by establishing work-capacity limits.

One method to help discuss the ease of access and ease of performance issues with patients is to have them fill out a brief activity profile. Clinicians can then review patients' answers and discuss with them their options. An example of an activity profile is shown in Table 1.

HELPING PATIENTS MAINTAIN THEIR MOTIVATION

After beginning an exercise program, the challenge is staying with it. Here are a few tips on helping patients maintain their motivation.

Encourage patients to "play smart." The smart athlete reduces or avoids downtime by training to avoid injuries. This involves proper stretching and warming up before exercise. It also means using proper equipment, especially footwear. Most important, patients need to avoid the temptation to do too much too fast: a gradual buildup is essential.

TABLE 1. *Activity Profile*

1. My typical day includes:

    ____ hours of sleep
    ____ hours of low activity (driving, reading, watching TV, etc.)
    ____ hours of moderate activity (walking, gardening, housework, etc.)
    ____ hours of vigorous activity (aerobic exercise, heavy labor, competitive sports)

2. The activities I enjoy most are:

    _____

3. The activities I would like to learn are:

    _____

4. I see the following as obstacles to exercising:

    ____ time   ____ fear of hypoglycemia
    ____ age   ____ skills/coordination
    ____ money   ____ family support
    ____ arthritis   ____ pain during or after exercise
    ____ energy   ____ lack of facilities
    ____ boredom

It is equally important for patients to keep tabs on their diabetes and how their exercise affects it. In particular, patients need to understand that the increased utilization of glucose during exercise can result in hypoglycemia both during the activity and for several hours after its completion.

Therefore, make sure patients know the symptoms of hypoglycemia and how to treat it, and instruct them to always carry some form of carbohydrate during exercise sessions. Teach them how to make appropriate adjustments in their regimen to minimize hypoglycemia.

Encourage patients to set a schedule in advance and stick to it. One of the best ways to keep on track is to set an exercise schedule in advance. Habits are developed through practice. Setting a schedule will help patients avoid scheduling other, conflicting activities.

Moreover, a schedule helps avoid the "I'll do it later" phenomenon. A regular schedule will also help patients to more effectively adjust their regimen so that they gain better control of their diabetes.

Encourage patients to get a training partner. In many cases, having an exercise partner helps one to start and continue an exercise plan. If a training partner is not a family member, counsel patients to discuss their diabetes with their partner, including what to do if they experience hypoglycemia.

Encourage patients to set realistic goals. It's important that the goals patients select are precisely defined and realistically attainable. Define goals by exercise *behavior* (e.g., walk for 30 minutes three times a week) rather than by an *outcome* of exercise (e.g., lose 20 pounds). Encourage patients to set a series of smaller, step-wise goals for which they can observe success and progress.

Encourage self-rewards. Progressive rewards for reaching exercise goals can increase motivation to stay with the exercise program.

Identify alternative exercise activities to reduce boredom. Individuals who become bored with a single activity should cross-train, i.e., identify a list of several activities that will help them to remain active. The goal, after all, is to do some form of exercise.

Explain the difference between "failure" and "backsliding." For some, any deviation from a schedule or not meeting the expectations is viewed as failure. It is important to make patients understand and accept off days as part of any long-term exercise program. When patients do have off days, reinforce the idea that they are experiencing a temporary "backslide" and the expectation that they will get back on track as soon as possible. Remind patients to tackle the future, not to haggle over the past.

CONCLUSION

Helping patients with diabetes incorporate exercise into their daily routine is a significant challenge. We have provided some guidelines to help in this process. Finally, for periodic frustration at a patient's lack of success, take a deep breath and relax. Directing such frustration toward the patient will not help. Instead, try teaming up with the patient by offering to help solve the problem. Not only will this help a patient get back on track, but it will also enhance the provider-patient relationship in general.

BIBLIOGRAPHY

American College of Sports Medicine: *ACSM's Guidelines for Exercise Testing and Prescription.* 5th ed. Baltimore, MD, Williams & Wilkins, 1995

Campaign B, Lampman RM: *Exercise in the Clinical Management of Diabetes.* Champaign, IL, Human Kinetics, 1994

The American Diabetes Association Council on Exercise: *The Fitness Book for People With Diabetes.* Hornsby WG, Ed. Alexandria, VA, American Diabetes Association, 1994

Helping Patients Understand and Recognize Hypoglycemia

9

Linda Gonder-Frederick, PhD,
Daniel J. Cox, PhD, and William L.
Clarke, MD

INTRODUCTION

Our research group has studied hypoglycemia in patients with type I diabetes for the past 15 years. From this research, we have developed blood glucose awareness training (BGAT), which improves a patient's ability to recognize, avoid, and treat hypoglycemia. In this chapter, we discuss the problem of hypoglycemia and its psychosocial consequences, as well as hypoglycemic symptoms and hypoglycemic unawareness.

THE PROBLEM OF HYPOGLYCEMIA

Hypoglycemia occurs when glucose levels in the bloodstream drop too low to maintain normal body function. In type I diabetes, low blood glucose (less than 70 mg/dl) is caused by an excess of insulin relative to food intake and/or physical activity.

Hypoglycemic episodes can be classified as *mild* or *severe* as shown in Table 1. These classifications are not based on any particular blood glucose (BG) level, but rather on 1) whether severe neuroglycopenia occurs and 2) whether or not the patient is able to self-treat. Neuroglycopenia occurs when glucose levels in the brain and central nervous system are too low to maintain normal function.

TABLE 1. *Hypoglycemic Episodes*

Mild

◆ Symptoms can include shaking, sweating, and slowed thinking
◆ Symptoms disappear with treatment
◆ Patient can self-treat

Severe

◆ Severe neuroglycopenic symptoms (lethargy, mental stupor, unconsciousness)
◆ Patient unable to self-treat and needs help from others

It is impossible to say that severe hypoglycemia occurs at any specific BG level, because individual patients respond very differently to low BG levels. Some patients become very symptomatic at BG levels of 60 mg/dl, while others show few symptoms at BG levels below 50 mg/dl. It is important for individual patients to know how *vulnerable* they are to symptoms at different low BG levels.

It is also important to emphasize that the term mild does not mean that these hypoglycemic episodes are inconsequential or that patients are only experiencing mild symptoms. It simply means that the patient did not become *so severely* neuroglycopenic that he or she was unable to self-treat. From the patient's perspective, even mild hypoglycemic episodes can be quite aversive and cause unpleasant symptoms, disruptions in ongoing activities, and social embarrassment.

Almost all patients taking insulin experience mild hypoglycemic episodes periodically. And, even though hypoglycemia is typically more problematic for type I patients, it is important to remember that it can occur in any patient taking BG-lowering medication.

Severe hypoglycemic episodes are more rare. However, there are many patients who have frequent and recurrent episodes, and even one episode can be traumatic and potentially dangerous. If severe hypoglycemia occurs, for example, when patients are performing critical tasks—such as driving a car, caring for children, operating dangerous equipment, or giving an important presentation at work—there can be serious negative consequences.

Obviously, a severe hypoglycemic episode can easily place the patient in physically dangerous and life-threatening situations. In fact, se-

T A B L E 2 . *Patients at High Risk for Fear of Hypoglycemia*

- ◆ Newly diagnosed patients who have not yet learned that they can deal effectively with hypoglycemia
- ◆ Patients who have had a recent or past traumatic episode
- ◆ Patients who tend to be overly anxious in other areas of their lives
- ◆ Parents of children who have experienced severe hypoglycemia or episodes while alone

vere hypoglycemia is the fourth leading cause of death in patients with type I diabetes.

FEAR OF HYPOGLYCEMIA

It is not all that surprising that many patients have considerable fear and anxiety about the possibility of hypoglycemia and its negative consequences. Sometimes this fear can result in inappropriate self-treatment, such as behaviors that keep BG in a higher, "safer" range. Table 2 lists patients who are at high risk for developing fear of hypoglycemia.

Whenever a patient has a traumatic experience with hypoglycemia, assess the patient's anxiety about a reoccurrence and the impact this has on his or her diabetes management. Ask the patient a few simple questions to assess fear, as shown in Table 3.

Family members and friends can also develop fear of hypoglycemia. Parents who have a young child with diabetes often show very high levels of fear, especially when the child has experienced unconsciousness due to hypoglycemia or had an episode when the parent was not present.

In both children and adults, fear of hypoglycemia can create tension and conflict in relationships. For example, after a traumatic episode, spouses or parents can become overprotective and hypervigilant, which is often resented by the patient.

HYPOGLYCEMIC SYMPTOMS

There are two primary methods for detecting hypoglycemia: 1) self-testing of BG and 2) feeling physical symptoms. Most patients typi-

TABLE 3. *Questions To Assess Fear of Hypoglycemia*

1. If there has been a recent or past traumatic experience, ask:
- How frightening/distressing was the episode for you?
- What negative consequences did the episode have (accidents, embarrassment, etc.)?
- Have you made any changes in your diabetes management to avoid another episode? (Look for behaviors that keep BG higher.)

2. Even if there has been no recent or past traumatic experience, ask:
- How much do you worry about having a hypoglycemic episode?
- How well do you think you are prepared to deal with a hypoglycemic episode?
- How do you make sure you will not become hypoglycemic during critical times, such as when driving or going to an important meeting? (Look for behaviors that keep BG higher.)

cally measure their BG only a few times each day. Therefore, the majority of hypoglycemic episodes occurs when patients are not doing a self-test or when their testing equipment is not available. For this reason, patients strongly rely on symptoms to tell them when their BG is too low.

Most hypoglycemic symptoms fall into one of two categories—autonomic or neuroglycopenic. Autonomic symptoms are those that have historically been considered the classic early warning signs; for example, trembling, sweating, and heart palpitations.

Most autonomic symptoms are caused by the hormonal counterregulation that occurs in response to low BG. Epinephrine secretion, which raises BG by stimulating the liver to release its stored glucose, is the most important counterregulatory response in type I diabetes.

Over time, however, many patients develop a decrease in their epinephrine response to low BG. This has the unfortunate effect of reducing the intensity of autonomic symptoms or delaying their onset.

Recent research shows that ability to counterregulate should be viewed as a continuum rather than as an "all or none" phenomenon. Counterregulation and the intensity of autonomic symptoms vary greatly among individual patients and within each individual patient across different times and situations. This is because counterregulation may be affected by many factors, including caffeine and alcohol consumption, recent low BG levels (see Chapter 10), the level of

TABLE 4. *Patients at High Risk for Decreased Counterregulation and Autonomic Symptoms*

Patients who

- ◆ Are in good glycemic control
- ◆ Are using intensive therapy
- ◆ Have autonomic neuropathy
- ◆ Experience frequent low BG levels
- ◆ Consume alcohol

Inform patients that alcohol can dampen their warning symptoms for hypoglycemia, as well as interfere with their body's ability to respond to hypoglycemia through decreased gluconeogenesis.

glycemic control, and autonomic neuropathy. Table 4 summarizes patient groups who are at high risk for decreased autonomic symptoms due to deficits in counterregulation.

Patients are typically not taught much about neuroglycopenic symptoms. Nor are they encouraged to use them as early warning cues. This is because neuroglycopenia was traditionally believed to occur only with extreme hypoglycemia, when patients were believed to be too stuporous to treat themselves.

We now know that neuroglycopenia can occur with even mild hypoglycemia, and that patients can recognize the subtle impairments that occur in their mental abilities with early neuroglycopenia.

Symptoms of mild neuroglycopenia include difficulty concentrating, slowed thinking, lightheadedness or dizziness, and uncoordination.

We recommend that clinicians encourage patients to use neuroglycopenic symptoms as early warning signs of hypoglycemia. To do this, have patients monitor their ability to think and perform routine tasks, then compare their current performance to their *usual* ability to do the tasks. For example, patients may notice that they have to exert more effort to follow a conversation or perform simple tasks, such as counting money. Patients can also do specific tasks or self-tests (mental subtractions, flipping a coin) to test their performance when they think they might be getting low.

Neuroglycopenic symptoms can be especially valuable as warning cues for patients who have decreased autonomic symptoms. Table 5 lists questions to help patients detect the early signs of neuroglycopenia.

TABLE 5. *Questions Patients Can Use to Check Themselves for Neuroglycopenia*

Compared to my usual ability to do this:

- ◆ Is it taking more effort to perform this task?
- ◆ Does this task seem more difficult than usual?
- ◆ Am I performing this task more slowly?
- ◆ Am I making more mistakes?
- ◆ In general, how impaired do I feel?

The degree to which individual patients experience neuroglycopenia with hypoglycemia varies greatly. Some patients become quite symptomatic with mild hypoglycemia, while others show few signs of neuroglycopenia even with BG levels of 45 mg/dl.

Obviously, patients who are extremely vulnerable to neuroglycopenia need to try to avoid any BG levels less than 70 mg/dl. One way to assess a patient's vulnerability is to review BG diaries and to question the patient carefully about any possible neuroglycopenic symptoms during BG readings below 70 mg/dl.

HYPOGLYCEMIA AND MOOD CHANGES

In addition to physical symptoms and disruptions in mental/motor abilities, many patients experience mood changes with hypoglycemia. These can range from feelings of anxiety and irritability, most likely caused by epinephrine secretion, to feelings of giddiness, most likely caused by neuroglycopenia.

Hypoglycemia tends to intensify moods that are already occurring. For this reason, patients need to monitor themselves for mood changes and emotional responses that seem *out of proportion* to whatever event is occurring.

Again, individual patients differ greatly in their tendency to experience mood changes with hypoglycemia. Some patients may just feel a little more tense than usual, while others, as described by one patient's husband, "can get downright belligerent."

Sometimes, positive moods occur with hypoglycemia, but usually the emotional changes are negative. Thus, it is easy to see how mood changes caused by hypoglycemia can create interpersonal tension, embarrassment, and even conflict. One of our patients, for example, reported that she had often been embarrassed by the "evil twin who appears" when she is hypoglycemic.

The stress that hypoglycemia-related mood changes can place on relationships is often clinically neglected. Again, help patients identify these problems by asking a few direct, but nonjudgmental, questions (e.g., Does hypoglycemia have any affect on your emotions or your moods? Have these emotional changes ever caused you to have problems, like arguments, with others?).

RECOGNIZING HYPOGLYCEMIC SYMPTOMS

Both epinephrine secretion and neuroglycopenia can cause a variety of different physical symptoms. While it is impossible to develop an exhaustive list of all hypoglycemic symptoms, Table 6 lists some of the most common ones. Patients typically do not experience all of these symptoms with hypoglycemia, and all patients do not experience the same symptoms. Hypoglycemic symptoms tend to be quite idiosyncratic. This means that the most reliable symptoms for one patient will not be the most reliable for another patient. For this reason, it is critical for patients to identify their own best warning symptoms.

Although most patients will report that they know what symptoms signal hypoglycemia for them, this is not always true. There are three psychological barriers to accurate symptom perception:

1. Inattentiveness
2. Inaccurate symptom beliefs
3. Misattribution of symptoms

Inattentiveness occurs when the patient is distracted, attending to a competing demand, or intensely focused on a task. Patients can also actively avoid paying attention to symptoms because they do not want to interrupt an enjoyable activity or have to ask others for help to find food.

Encourage all patients to monitor their symptoms carefully, especially at those times when their BG is more likely to be low (when insulin is peaking, less food has been eaten, or physical activity has increased).

TABLE 6. *Symptoms of Hypoglycemia*

Autonomic	Neuroglycopenic	Mood Changes
Trembling/Shaking	Slow Thinking	Nervous/Tense
Pounding Heart	Lightheaded/Dizziness	Jittery
Fast Pulse	Trouble Concentrating	Irritated
Flushed Face	Slurred Speech	Worried
Sweating	Blurred Vision	Frustrated
Temperature Changes	Difficulty Reading	Angry
Queasy Stomach	or Talking	Distressed
Weakness	Sleepiness	Sad/Unhappy
Tingling (extremities)	Numbness	Stubborn
Headache	Uncoordination	Giddy
Heavy Breathing		Euphoric

Some patients tend to attribute any symptom they experience to their diabetes. This can result in inaccurate or "false alarm" symptom beliefs. These are symptoms that patients believe are reliable signs of hypoglycemia but that are, in reality, independent of BG. Symptoms that tend to be false alarms are hunger and fatigue, which are just as likely to occur with normal or high BG levels.

Patients can also misattribute symptoms that are related to hypoglycemia to some other cause. For example, a patient playing softball may think that his or her sweating is due to exercising in the heat rather than hypoglycemia. A patient facing an important work deadline may attribute a sudden feeling of nervousness to stress.

Because symptom perception is not always accurate, we recommend that clinicians *objectively* assess which symptoms are the most reliable cues for individual patients. In blood glucose awareness training (BGAT), patients do this by keeping a BG diary that requires them to "scan" themselves for symptoms, then record these before testing their BG. The clinician and patient then review the diary and simply count the number of times each symptom occurred with BG levels 1) below 70 mg/dl and 2) greater than 120 mg/dl. This gives a measure of 1) how *sensitive* the symptom is to hypoglycemia and 2) how *specific* the symptom is to hypoglycemia, respectively.

The best symptoms are those that are both sensitive and specific, i.e., they occur most of the time that BG is low and rarely when BG is not low. Repeat this type of symptom assessment when patients report a change in their symptoms or an increased frequency of asymptomatic hypoglycemia. Chapter 10 provides more techniques for using similar diaries to assess and improve BG detection.

HYPOGLYCEMIC UNAWARENESS

Some patients experience a reduction or loss of autonomic hypoglycemic symptoms over time. As we have previously noted, this can be caused by a number of factors—some of them transitory (e.g., alcohol consumption) and some of them permanent (e.g., autonomic neuropathy).

There is now evidence that hypoglycemic unawareness is reversible: autonomic symptoms increase when patients raise their average BG level and meticulously avoid low BG. Unfortunately, this strategy can also jeopardize metabolic control. For this reason, we recommend that clinicians first rule out the possibility that the patient has symptoms that they are not attending to or using optimally.

In our research, we have found that even patients who are classified as hypoglycemic unaware actually have some symptoms that reliably covary with their low BG. Furthermore, we have shown that patients presumed to be hypoglycemic unaware improve their ability to detect hypoglycemia when they undergo BGAT. For these reasons, we think of hypoglycemic awareness/unawareness as a continuum and use the term "reduced hypoglycemic awareness" to describe patients having problems recognizing symptoms.

When patients report reduced awareness of hypoglycemic symptoms, have them follow the BG diary procedure described in the previous section. This will help to identify reliable symptoms and often increases patient attentiveness to symptoms as well. Teach and encourage these patients to use mild neuroglycopenic symptoms as early warning signs of hypoglycemia.

CONCLUSION

Hypoglycemic episodes are a major problem for many insulin-taking patients. In addition to placing patients at physical risk, hypoglycemia can have serious psychological consequences. These include extreme fear of hypoglycemia and conflicts in relationships. Patients rely on symptoms to warn them that their BG is too low. Because both the type and intensity of hypoglycemic symptoms vary from patient to patient, it is important to help patients identify their own best warning cues. In addition to the "classic" autonomic symptoms (trembling, sweating), patients need to be taught to monitor neuroglycopenic symptoms and mood changes. Clinicians can objectively assess patients' symptoms by using a simple BG diary in which patients record their symptoms along with their BG self-tests. Patients who may benefit from this type of assessment include those who report a decrease in their hypoglycemic symptoms and those who have problems with recurrent severe hypoglycemic episodes.

ACKNOWLEDGMENTS

This work was supported, in part, by grants from the National Institutes of Health (R01-DK-28288 and RR-00847).

BIBLIOGRAPHY

Cox DJ, Gonder-Frederick LA, Antoun B, Cryer PE, Clarke WL: Perceived symptoms in the recognition of hypoglycemia. *Diabetes Care* 16:519–527, 1993

Gonder-Frederick LA, Cox DJ, Driesen NR, Ryan CM, Clarke WL: Individual differences in neurobehavioral disruption during mild and moderate hypoglycemia in adults with IDDM. *Diabetes* 43:1407–1412, 1994

Irvine A, Cox D, Gonder-Frederick L: Fear of hypoglycemia: relationship to glycemic control and psychological factors in IDDM patients. *Health Psychol* 11:135–138, 1992

Helping Patients Reduce Severe Hypoglycemia | 10

Daniel J. Cox, PhD,
Linda Gonder-Frederick, PhD, and
William L. Clarke, MD

INTRODUCTION

S evere hypoglycemia can lead to multiple negative consequences, such as automobile accidents, social embarrassment, and lost employment. The occurrence of severe hypoglycemia increases as metabolic control improves. Fear of having an insulin reaction can discourage patients from pursuing improved metabolic control. However, there are some simple steps that can be taken to avoid this problem.

NATURE OF LOW BLOOD GLUCOSE EVENTS

In order to help patients avoid severe hypoglycemia, there are four general points to keep in mind: 1) anticipate low blood glucose, 2) avoid low blood glucose, 3) recognize low blood glucose, and 4) know how to treat low blood glucose.

Low blood glucose is defined as blood glucose (BG) less than 70 mg/dl. There are four reasons to avoid low BG:

1. **Frequent low BG significantly increases the risk of severe hypoglycemia.** "If you play with fire, you're likely to get burnt." In a recent study, subjects whose home BG diaries consisted of more than 12% low BG readings, compared with subjects who had fewer than 12%, were four times more likely to experience severe hypoglycemia

TABLE 1. *Avoid Low BG (Less Than 70 mg/dl) Because*

1. It increases the risk of severe hypoglycemia.
2. It increases the risk of recurrent low BG.
3. It reduces low BG autonomic symptoms in the next 48 hours.
4. Nocturnal low BG can lead to severe hypoglycemia.

over the next 6 months. Consequently, if a patient is having frequent low BG readings, try altering his or her insulin regimen.

2. **Low BG leads to recurrent low BG.** During the first 24 hours following a low BG episode, patients have a 50% chance, on average, of having a repeat low BG episode. This probability falls to 25% over the next 24 hours and progressively declines after that. Consequently, if a patient has low BG, he or she may want to slightly increase carbohydrate intake, reduce long-acting insulin, or measure BG more often over the subsequent 24 hours.

3. **Recurrent low BG results in fewer autonomic symptoms.** Patients might want to measure their BG more often after a low BG episode because the next 24 to 48 hours will, in general, be associated with fewer autonomic symptoms. The opposite of this is also true—patients who complain of reduced warning symptoms of hypoglycemia may become symptomatic again if they avoid frequent low BG events (Table 1).

4. **Nocturnal low BG can progress to severe hypoglycemia.** Low BG occurring while patients sleep can go undetected and progress "silently" until a seizure occurs. It is far better to prevent nocturnal low BG than risk severe hypoglycemia.

PREVENTION

To avoid low BG, patients need to know and appropriately apply information about peak insulin action, carbohydrate metabolism, and the impact of exercise and self-care routines (Table 2).

Insulin

Select an insulin regimen that best fits the patient's metabolism and lifestyle. This will typically involve having the patient take different

TABLE 2. *Things to Know and Apply to Avoid Hypoglycemia*

Insulin Action

◆ When insulin action is peaking
◆ When insulin action is at its nadir
◆ When to eat
◆ When to exercise
◆ Effects of changing injection time

Food

◆ Carbohydrates raise BG in 30 to 60 minutes.
◆ Fat slows metabolism.
◆ Protein has a minimal effect on BG.
◆ Glucose raises BG in 15 to 20 minutes.
◆ Carbohydrates should peak before insulin peaks.

Exercise

◆ Any increased activity above routine can affect BG.
◆ Exercise plus high insulin, BG falls quickly.
◆ Exercise plus very low insulin, BG may rise.

Self-Care Routine

◆ Low BG is frequently caused by disruptions in routine.
◆ Patient's metabolism and lifestyle may be differentially sensitive to disruptions in insulin, food, and/or exercise.
◆ Keep diaries to identify sensitivity.

---

types of insulin at different times. The effects of long- and short-acting insulins overlap. Patients need to know when these combined insulins are most and least active. Knowing this will help them better anticipate when to look for signs of hypoglycemia and hyperglycemia, when to and when not to eat and exercise, and what to expect if they take their insulin earlier or later than usual. Most patients have no idea how their different insulins combine to produce peak insulin action.

Food

Patients need to know that it is primarily carbohydrates that raise BG, and that most carbohydrates do not begin to have their maximum effects on BG for 30 to 60 minutes after eating. The only exceptions to this are glucose, which raises BG within 15 to 20 minutes, and high-fat meals (e.g., over 40% fat), which may delay carbohydrate absorption. This information is important in order to match food intake with anticipated insulin peaks. If the insulin peaks before the carbohydrates, then the patient is at increased risk of hypoglycemia. Assess patients' knowledge by determining whether they know the latest they can eat, given their peak insulin actions, and when to eat snacks. Help patients avoid hypoglycemia by correcting any misconceptions and coming to a mutual understanding about when and what they need to eat.

Exercise

Many people believe they exercise only when they put on sneakers and go to the gym. They do not appreciate that any increased level of physical activity over their routine represents a potential disruption in their insulin-food balance. They may also not realize that the effects of exercise depend on the amount of insulin in their system. While exercise at times of peak insulin action will send BG down quickly, the same exercise when insulin action is at its nadir may actually result in a BG rise. Consequently, patients must realize that increased physical activity beyond their routine level, at times when their insulin level is high and their BG level is near normal or lower, will increase the risk of hypoglycemia. Additionally, patients need to realize that prolonged intensive exercise can deplete glucose stores, making it difficult to raise BG with a routine carbohydrate snack after such exercise.

Self-Care Routine

We have reported that 85% of low BG episodes can be accounted for by disruptions in one's routine self-treatment behaviors: taking more insulin than usual, eating less than usual, or exercising more than usual. However, some individuals are more sensitive to disruptions in their insulin routine, while others are more affected by changes in their food intake, and still others are more affected by changes in activity level.

The only way for a patient to know whether his or her low BG levels are associated with changes in insulin, food, or exercise routines is by keeping a diary for several weeks. Before measuring BG, have the patient write in the diary (see Figure 1) whether he or she just had more, less, or the usual amount of food, insulin, or activity. Review the data and compare those times when BG was low/not low to see if there is any pattern relative to disruptions in self-care routines. Once a relationship is identified, counsel the patient to not overadjust insulin, to anticipate low BG when eating less than usual, or to eat more when engaging in nonroutine exercise.

RECOGNIZING LOW BG

Patients can recognize when they are low based on either symptoms or disruptions in their routine performance. Since patients experience low BG in different ways, the challenge is to help patients identify their best cues of low BG. The four most common symptoms of low BG are 1) pounding heart, 2) difficulty concentrating, 3) jittery, tense, or nervous, and 4) uncoordination. As mentioned in Chapter 9, there are three barriers to detecting symptoms of low BG: inattention, misinterpretation, and inaccurate symptom beliefs.

Disruptions in Performance

In addition to specific symptoms, have patients attend to disruptions in their routine performance. Since neuroglycopenia slows cognitive-motor performance, typists may notice low BG because their typing is slowing or is requiring more effort; the carpenter may find himself dropping more nails; the waitress may find it more difficult making change; the receptionist may find it more difficult following what someone is saying. These performance cues can be the earliest signs of low BG, and they are especially important for people who have lost their previously familiar signs of hypoglycemia.

Identifying Sensitive and Specific Low BG Cues

For any symptom or cue to be useful to a patient, it must be sensitive and specific. That is, it must occur frequently when BG is low, and it must occur rarely when BG is not low. For example, "hunger" is typically not a good cue of low BG because it is not specific to low BG, i.e., it occurs frequently when BG is not low. The best way to identify which cues are sensitive and specific is through systematic data collection. Using a diary, have patients routinely record their symptoms and disruptions in routine performance just before measuring their BG. After collecting 8 to 10 low BG readings, have patients review this data and identify 1) which cues were present when their BG was low and 2) which cues were not present when their BG was not low. Such cues represent sensitive and specific indicators of low BG. Typically, a good symptom is present more than 50% of the time when BG is low and less than 10% of the time when BG is not low.

Ability to Detect Low BG

Like symptoms, patients' beliefs about their ability to recognize low BG are not always accurate. It is important not only to recognize how accurate a patient is but also to enhance this accuracy. Again, the best way to address these issues is through systematic data collection in the patient's daily routine. Just before measuring BG, have the patient record a BG estimate in a diary. In reviewing these data, calculate the percentage of times the patient was low and recognized it (number of BG estimates less than 70 mg/dl when actual BG was low/number of actual BG levels less than 70 mg/dl). A good detection rate is over 50%. Identifying hypoglycemia unawareness may encourage more frequent use of home BG monitoring.

In order to improve detection of low BG, encourage patients to look for, and deliberately use, those cues found to be sensitive and specific. Have patients reevaluate their situation whenever their BG was low and they did not recognize it. Whenever this happens, have the patient ask himself or herself:

- What subtle cues did I miss?
- Why didn't I notice them?
- Was I performing differently from usual?
- Was my insulin, food, and exercise different from routine?
- How active was my insulin?
- Have I had low BG in the past 24 to 48 hours?

After systematically asking and answering such questions, have the patient record these "missed opportunities" in the diary and consider them in the future (Table 3).

TABLE 3. *Recognition of Low BG*

Disruptions in Performance

◆ Look for slowed, more difficult performance.
◆ Occur at same BG level as autonomic symptoms.
◆ Are important if autonomic symptoms lost.

BG Estimation Accuracy

◆ Record estimated and actual BG.
◆ Calculate % detected.
◆ Greater than 50% detection is good.

Ability to Detect Low BG

◆ Patients frequently overestimate ability.
◆ Use diaries to determine how accurate and when inaccurate.
◆ When inaccurate, review missed opportunities.

TREATING LOW BG

Counsel patients to treat low BG as soon as they recognize it. Waiting until they have driven to work, gotten the kids off to school, their visitor has left, or the symptoms have gotten worse only makes treating it more difficult. Unfortunately, patients often delay treating low BG because of a sense of embarrassment, a feeling of failure or weakness, or the hassles of stopping what they are doing. Make sure patients are fully aware of the potential costs associated with not treating their low BG, such as possibly losing their driver's license.

After patients decide to treat, the next decision is what to treat with and how much. We strongly encourage our patients to routinely carry prepackaged commercial glucose in the same way they carry their watch or driver's license, i.e., to keep it readily available in a known location, so that when patients are low they do not have to work very hard to get to this glucose. We encourage commercial glucose, because

- Glucose raises BG quickly.
- It is prepackaged and not alluring, discouraging overtreatment.
- Consuming it is inconspicuous.
- It stores easily and reliably.

The general guidelines for taking glucose tablets, assuming 5 grams of carbohydrates/tablet, are

TABLE 4. *Treatment Issues*

1. Treat immediately.

2. Don't overtreat.

3. Treat with glucose.

4. Follow treatment with:

   Food to keep BG up.
   Self-monitoring of BG at 15 to 20 minutes after treatment.

- If BG is 65 to 80 mg/dl and there is no immediate meal, take 2 tablets.
- If BG is less than 65 mg/dl, take 3 to 4 tablets.
- Test BG 15 to 20 minutes after treatment.
- Repeat treatment until BG rises above 85 mg/dl.
- Since carbohydrates keep BG up for only about 60 minutes, eat additional food to keep BG up.

Patients frequently use low BG as an opportunity to eat those foods they would otherwise avoid, such as cookies. This is undesirable, because such foods frequently have large amounts of fat, do not raise BG as quickly as glucose, and are frequently overeaten (Table 4).

A SAMPLE BG DIARY

The sample BG diary in Figure 1 can be used to help identify self-care behaviors that increase the risk of low BG, clarify cues that herald the presence of low BG, determine the patient's ability to detect low BG, and identify "missed opportunities." The sample diary can be copied for patient use. Instructions for its use appear at the bottom of the diary. For this diary to be useful, have patients fill it out until they have had 8 to 10 low BG readings. It may be helpful to have patients color-code entries when BG was low in order to easily compare them with entries when BG was not low. This can easily be reduced to percentages: the percentage of times the symptom occurred, the performance cue was detected, extra insulin was used, meals were skipped, etc. Formalized blood glucose awareness training (BGAT) provides patients with a systematic approach to enhance anticipation, prevention, awareness, and treatment of low BG.

FIGURE 1. BG Diary Sheet

Cues: Scan your body for dryness in mouth and nose or changes in your: thinking, vision, taste, balance, sweating, breathing, heart rate, coordination, urination, hunger, energy, tension, tolerance, insulin, food, activity, others.

BG Diary Sheet

Name: _____

Date	Time	I	F	E	Symptoms and Performance Cues	Est	Actual	Missed	Opportunities/Treatment

First, list the date and time of each entry. I, F, and E refer to your most recent insulin, food, and exercise. In each of these columns, write M, L, or U if you took more, less, or your usual amount of insulin, food, and exercise. Next, write in any BG cues you might have, including any symptoms, disruptions in routine performance, time of day, whether you recently had low BG, whether your insulin is peaking, etc. Based on these BG cues, estimate your BG and write that in the Est column. Next, measure and record your actual BG in the Actual column. If your BG was low (less than 70 mg/dl) and you did not recognize this, ask yourself, "What cues did I miss and why?" Write down the cues you missed in the Missed column and why you missed them in the Opportunities/Treatment column.

After 30 to 50 entries, take a yellow marker and highlight all those times when your actual BG was less than 70 mg/dl. When your BG was low, were you more likely to take more insulin, eat less, or exercise more compared to when you were not low? What symptoms occurred only when you were low? What percent of the time did you recognize when you were low? When you failed to recognize low BG, what cues did you miss that you can look for in the future?

CONCLUSION

Arming patients with knowledge and providing them with the learning experience of BG diaries can significantly aid in patients' awareness and understanding about how their bodies respond to hypoglycemia. With this, patients who are vulnerable to severe hypoglycemia can learn to reduce the occurrence of such events.

ACKNOWLEDGMENTS

This study was supported in part by grants from the National Institutes of Health (RO1-DK-28288 and RR-00847). The authors thank the invaluable assistance of Ms. Diana Jullian.

BIBLIOGRAPHY

Cox D, Gonder-Frederick L, Polonsky W, Schlundt D, Julian D, Clarke W: A multicenter evaluation of blood glucose awareness training—II. *Diabetes Care* 18:523–528, 1995

COMPLEX AND CHRONIC BEHAVIORAL ISSUES

The results of the DCCT and other studies underline the important protective effects of tight blood glucose control for people with type I diabetes. Yet, it is extraordinarily difficult for most people to achieve near-normal blood glucose levels and to maintain them over long periods of time. In his chapter, Jacobson offers guidelines for determining effective strategies to improve glycemic control among patients who have type I diabetes. He emphasizes the point that any improvement in glycemia is associated with a reduced risk of diabetes-related complications. Jacobson goes on to discuss the advantages and disadvantages of a gradual approach and a more rapid radical approach to achieving the goal of improved glycemia, and he offers suggestions for effectively pursuing each approach.

Wing reminds us that weight loss is a key component in the management of obese individuals with type II diabetes, that it helps in the prevention of diabetes in those with impaired glucose tolerance, and that it is important in the prevention and/or treatment of weight gain in people with type I diabetes using intensive insulin therapy. Yet most clinicians have had limited success in their efforts to help patients with diabetes lose weight. Some have even given up trying. Wing's chapter provides information and strategies to help patients see that it is possible to succeed in weight loss.

Fisher, Ziff, and Haire-Joshu discuss the often underappreciated issue of smoking and diabetes. They point out that the cardiovascular risks when a person with diabetes smokes are as high as 14 times those of either smoking or diabetes alone. Smoking is also associated with an increased incidence of other diabetes complications, including neuropathy and arterial occlusive disease. Yet the prevalence of smoking among adults with diabetes may be higher than among the population at large, and the rate of smoking cessation may be lower among those with diabetes. The authors offer a set of practical guidelines for encouraging smoking cessation among patients who have diabetes.

A drive for thinness is endemic among many adolescents and young women in our society, and this drive does not appear to be reduced among those who have diabetes. In fact, the emphasis on diet and weight control, which is a fact of life for people with diabetes, only heightens this preoccupation for many. Studies conducted over the past 15 years among young women with type I diabetes show the destructive consequences of eating-disordered behavior in terms of metabolic derangement and a consequent increased risk of diabetes-related complications. In their chapter, Rapaport, LaGreca, and Levine offer a model for preventing eating disorders in young women with diabetes. The authors discuss why eating disorders develop and suggest strategies for primary prevention.

Depression in people with diabetes is a prevalent, chronic condition, with consequences beyond its recognized effects on mental functioning. As Lustman, Griffith, and Clouse point out, depression complicates the medical management of diabetes by influencing the reporting of diabetes symptoms, regimen adherence, glycemic control, and the risk of long-term complications. The authors offer suggestions for treating depression in patients with diabetes, emphasizing the importance of effective treatment for improving mood, glycemic control, and overall quality of life.

Improving Glycemic Control in Patients With Type I Diabetes

11

Alan M. Jacobson, MD

INTRODUCTION

The results of the Diabetes Control and Complications Trial (DCCT) and other studies have underlined the important protective benefit of normalizing blood glucose levels over long periods of time in patients with type I diabetes.

A direct and generally linear relationship between level of glycemic control and progression of complications has been found. Thus, modest improvement of glycemia can lead to modest improvement in medical outcomes. Moreover, improving glycemia to levels that are close to the nondiabetic range can dramatically reduce the risk of complications.

The majority of patients, even under ideal circumstances, face a daunting challenge when the goal is optimal regulation of glycemia. Indeed, only 5% of patients in the DCCT, a carefully selected and closely monitored group of patients enrolled in a research protocol, maintained HbA_{1c} levels in the normal, nondiabetic range through the whole trial.

The good news, that substantial improvement in glycemia lowers the risk of complications, is balanced by the bad news, that it's very hard to accomplish. This makes optimal diabetes care a behavioral, psychosocial, and motivational challenge for clinicians and patients. This chapter offers suggestions for strategies in the evaluation and care of diabetic patients when improving glycemic control is the objective.

CHOOSE AN APPROACH FOR CHANGE

Two different broad approaches can be used when improved glycemia is the goal: 1) gradual, modest change and 2) rapid, radical change. There is no specific research evidence to suggest that either approach works better in improving glycemic control. It is best to consider the advantages and disadvantages of each for each patient.

In practice, clinicians often take the former approach, successively introducing small changes in regimen to the patient. This may be selected because it is more feasible in many practice settings. In principle, this allows the patient to make modest adjustments to increasingly demanding therapeutic goals, e.g., increasing the number of insulin injections and frequency of testing, using algorithms, making dietary alterations, and modifying activities over time. This may also have the benefit of helping the patient build self-confidence, thereby allowing him or her to gradually take on more demanding aspects of therapy.

While this approach allows the patient to gradually adapt the treatment regimen to his or her current lifestyle, it may never give the patient the opportunity to fully experience intensive treatment, because the educational and motivational approach never clearly emphasizes this large step.

The alternative approach of thorough initial education, together with rapid initiation of an intensive protocol, supported by close, careful medical follow-up, may enhance the achievement of normalized blood glucose levels. However, this immersion strategy requires considerable education over a short time frame and frequent contact with members of the treatment team to learn and implement each element of the new therapeutic regimen.

Because the patient may feel overwhelmed by the drastic changes in treatment, the support of an available treatment team is critical during the initiation phase. Ideally, the health-care team can discuss both approaches with the patient and allow the patient to make decisions about more radical versus gradual change in therapy.

FOSTER A COOPERATIVE HEALTH-CARE TEAM

To make the goal of normalized glycemic control feasible for patients typically requires participation from all members of the health-care team, including the physician, nurse, dietitian, exercise physiologist, and mental health professional. Periodic meetings of team members will likely help solidify a collaborative approach.

EVALUATE PATIENTS

Evaluate patients carefully to select treatment and strategies, identify educational and motivational needs, assess barriers to success, and determine which approach to improving glycemia is best. The evaluation process is an opportunity for the patient to consider less intensive approaches. In that sense, a careful evaluation can help clinicians design a treatment regimen whether or not rapid intensification is the specific approach taken.

Begin with a thorough understanding of the patient's personal circumstances, including financial resources, sources of emotional support, environmental stresses, history of psychiatric illness, attitudes toward weight and diet, psychological adjustment to diabetes, and sources of motivation for change. Intense concerns about weight and weight gain and strong worries about hypoglycemia are particularly important psychosocial barriers to intensification. Be aware that none of these personal and social characteristics is absolutely predictive of the patient's ability to change or to implement intensive diabetes management strategies. Rather, an examination of these generic and diabetes-specific psychosocial issues allows clinician and patient to jointly explore the new treatment and its place in the patient's life.

Specific measures, such as the Problem Areas in Diabetes (PAID) and the Diabetes Quality of Life (DQOL) can help identify areas of patient concern and worry and thereby serve as aids to assessment.

It is also instructive to involve an important person in the patient's life, e.g., the spouse, a child, a parent, or a close friend, in the evaluation. Assessment of the patient's views of diabetes as seen through the eyes of an important other person often reveals issues that can be incorporated in planning intensive therapy.

IMPLEMENT A BRIEF TRIAL

Consider a small dose of intensive treatment as a guide to planning therapy. In general, the best predictor of future action is past action. Thus, patients with a recent history of serious adherence problems in care of diabetes are less likely to withstand the rigors of full intensification.

When given the opportunity to make changes in diabetes care, patients often have idealized expectations. Therefore, it is useful to give them a small dose of intensive treatment before making final decisions for a major change in goals.

In the DCCT, a 2-week period of behavioral tasks that included modification of testing frequency and careful recording of activities was used to help the patient decide about entering the study in light of his or her experience. In the DCCT, changes in the actual insulin regimen could not be made to ensure proper randomization.

In clinical practice, behavioral tasks can include trying a lunchtime injection of regular insulin, based on prelunch glucose results, or trying out an algorithm for the morning injection of regular insulin. These can help patients know a bit more about the actual work entailed.

Evaluation of the patient's personal reactions, sense of self-efficacy, and specific anticipated problem areas after such a brief trial can help the patient and provider plan therapy.

HELP PATIENTS MANAGE CHANGE

Recognize that each patient will require his or her own plan for intensification—one size does not fit all; furthermore, *changes in strategy are often required*. What may have started as an apparently straightforward request for intensification becomes a series of interactions in which the patient and provider change treatment. Even though the patient seems openly desirous of intensification, the patient may experience change as a loss. Even the most enthusiastic patient may back off from an agreed-upon plan when such losses become apparent. Intensification involves thinking about diabetes. Patients may discover that this intrudes too much on the day. This reaction may reflect the time demands faced by busy people. In addition, considering intensive diabetes care every day may lead to the sudden thrusting of unpleasant realities into the awareness of someone who has not fully accepted the diabetes as a real part of his or her life.

Consult with a mental health professional to identify effective strategies to help patients deal with their feelings. There are many different approaches for psychosocial intervention; no single strategy can be depended on over long-term treatment of a chronic illness such as type I diabetes. For example, sometimes it may be most useful to help patients express and experience feelings. Other times specific behavioral plans may help patients adapt to the demands of intensification.

A mental health professional can present an array of possible therapeutic strategies that may vary from patient to patient and within a patient over time. Refer patients to a mental health professional to help implement or change the plan when, for example, 1) the patient's glycemic control is not improving, 2) the patient is openly struggling with feelings about intensified treatment, 3) the patient acknowledges openly that there are key impediments (such as family problems or work stress), or 4) the clinician is getting frustrated by the lack of change.

Note that the patient who has met the mental health professional in the assessment period is less likely to see such a referral in frightening terms. In essence, the social distance between the patient and the mental health professional has been decreased by an early exposure.

MANAGE PROVIDER FEELINGS

Intensive diabetes treatment demands more from providers as well as patients. In particular, intensive treatment necessitates a more intimate working relationship than conventional therapy. Weekly telephone contact, faxing, and e-mail will often lead to stronger personal relationships and to stronger feelings as well. In this context, patients are likely to reveal more personal, emotional information and also form more intense therapeutic bonds.

Intensified relationships may provoke strong feelings of various kinds. Neither the clinician nor the patient may be accustomed to the intensity of this involvement, because the typical pattern of care rarely exceeds three to four visits per year. Some of these feelings may complicate the treatment process. Patients may become unexpectedly dependent, provocative, or openly emotional. Clinicians may find their own feelings of bonding turning to frustration, or even to anger, depending on the patient's therapeutic course.

For example, a patient may initially seem like an ideal candidate for intensive treatment, but over several months, may fail to achieve significant change in glycemic control, thereby frustrating the clinician. This can cause disappointment and even anger. Alternatively, the patient may bring up unexpected and uncomfortable personal experiences because he or she is participating in a more intimate relationship.

Sharing may serve to make the therapeutic bond friendlier and more positive; it may also lead the patient to divulge information that the clinician finds uncomfortable. A skilled mental health professional, who has experience treating diabetic patients, can help the provider identify effective strategies for managing feelings that may arise in treating patients intensively (see Chapter 18).

CONCLUSION

The findings from the DCCT offer a positive message to patients with type I diabetes. However, current methods of intensive treatment require considerable medical, educational, and psychosocial skill for optimal implementation.

ACKNOWLEDGMENTS

Supported by National Institutes of Health Grants DK-42315 and DK-247845 and the Herbert Graetz Fund.

BIBLIOGRAPHY

The DCCT Research Group: Are continuing studies of metabolic control and microvascular complications in insulin-dependent diabetes mellitus justified? *N Engl J Med* 318:246–250, 1988

The DCCT Research Group: Influence of intensive diabetes treatment on quality-of-life outcomes in the Diabetes Control and Complications Trial. *Diabetes Care* 19:195–203, 1996

Jacobson AM: Medically unexplained symptoms: the diagnosis and therapeutic approach to somatoform and factitious disorders and malingering. In *Psychiatric Secrets*. Jacobson JL, Jacobson AM, Eds. Philadelphia, PA, Hanley and Belfus, 1996

Jacobson AM: Psychological considerations in the care of patients with insulin-dependent diabetes mellitus. *N Engl J Med*. In press

Jacobson AM, de Groot M, Samson JA: The evaluation of two measures of quality of life in patients with type I and type II diabetes mellitus. *Diabetes Care* 17:267–274, 1994

Jacobson AM, Hauser S, Anderson B, Polonsky W: Psychosocial aspects of diabetes. In *Joslin's Diabetes Mellitus*. 13th ed. Kahn C, Weir G, Eds. Philadelphia, PA, Lea & Febiger, 1994

Kaplan SH, Greenfield S, Ware JE: Assessing the effects of physician-patient interactions on the outcomes of chronic disease. *Med Care* 27:S110–S127, 1989

Lipkin M, Putnam S, Lazare A: *The Medical Interview: Clinical Care, Education, and Research*. New York, Springer-Verlag, 1995

Polonsky W, Anderson B, Welch G, Jacobson A: Assessment of diabetes-specific distress. *Diabetes Care* 18:754–760, 1995

Improving Weight Loss and Maintenance in Patients With Diabetes

12

Rena R. Wing, PhD

INTRODUCTION

Weight loss is important for patients with diabetes. It is a key component in the management of obese patients with type II diabetes, helps in the prevention of diabetes in those with impaired glucose tolerance, and is important in the prevention and/or treatment of weight gain in patients with type I diabetes who are using intensive insulin therapy.

However, long-term results of most weight control programs are disappointing, and thus, many clinicians have given up even trying to help patients lose weight. This is an example of what psychologists call a self-fulfilling prophecy—if you think you are going to fail, it is very likely you will fail. So too, if patients embark on weight loss efforts with the expectation that they will be unable to lose weight or to maintain their loss, they are more likely to fail in their efforts.

This chapter provides information and strategies that may help convince clinicians and patients that it is possible to succeed in weight loss. Changing expectations is the first step in changing outcomes.

SET A REASONABLE GOAL OF LOSING 10% OF INITIAL WEIGHT

The average woman entering a weight-loss program for individuals with type II diabetes weighs 220 pounds. Looking at a Metropolitan

Life Insurance chart or other table of ideal body weight and telling this patient that she should weigh 140 pounds is a setup for failure. It is far more reasonable to aim for a weight loss of 10% of initial body weight (have the 220-pound woman try to lose 22 pounds and maintain it).

Such modest weight losses have been shown to produce long-term improvements in glycemic control. In a study of overweight patients with type II diabetes, subjects who lost 15 to 30 pounds and maintained it for a year had long-term improvement in HbA$_1$, insulin, HDL cholesterol, and triglycerides.

STRESS EXERCISE AS MUCH OR MORE THAN DIET

Exercise is the strongest predictor of long-term maintenance of weight loss. Programs that combine diet plus exercise achieve better long-term weight loss than programs stressing diet or exercise alone. Adding exercise to a diet program also minimizes the loss of lean body mass, improves the serum lipid profile, and produces better long-term improvements in glycemic control. Moreover, in studies comparing successful weight losers with those who relapse, the variable that best distinguishes these two groups is the amount of exercise performed.

In recommending exercise to a patient, it is important to set a goal that the patient can achieve. We recommend starting very slowly, i.e., encouraging the patient to just get out the door for a short walk (10 to 15 minutes) on 3 days each week. After the patient achieves this goal for a few weeks, then the distances can be gradually increased until the patient is walking 2 miles/day on 5 days/week.

The goal in weight-loss programs is to increase energy expenditure; this goal is best accomplished by increasing the distance walked rather than the speed (or intensity), since walking 1 mile and jogging 1 mile use a similar number of calories. A good rule to remember is the following: **walking 1 mile uses 100 calories**.

Thus, if a patient walks 10 miles each week, he or she will be using an extra 1,000 kcal of energy. Patients can also expend an additional 100 calories by riding a stationary bicycle for 15 to 30 minutes, raking leaves for 20 minutes, weight lifting for 30 minutes, or playing tennis for 15 minutes.

It is helpful to encourage patients to set aside a time each day for the purpose of exercise and also to try to increase exercise in their daily routine (such as using stairs instead of elevators). Encourage patients to record their exercise on a daily basis and total it for the week, the month, and the year. These totals help patients see the progress they are making.

PRESCRIBE A LOW-FAT/LOW-CALORIE DIET WITH SELF-MONITORING

Several recent studies have suggested that moderate calorie restriction, in combination with a low fat intake, may be the most effective dietary approach for weight loss. When subjects have been taught to limit fat intake only, with no restrictions placed on total calories, weight losses have been modest (2 to 3 kg). Better results have been achieved when both fat and calories were targeted.

In a recent study, type II subjects in the low-calorie/low-fat treatment group consumed 1,000 to 1,500 kcal, with 20% of calories from fat, and self-monitored calories and fat grams. Subjects in the other treatment group focused on calorie restriction only; these subjects ate 1,000 to 1,500 kcal/day and limited fat intake to less than 30% of calories. Because the emphasis in their program was on calorie restriction alone, subjects self-monitored calories only. Weight losses at the end of the 16-week program and at 1-year follow-up were better in subjects who focused on calories plus fat than in subjects who focused on calorie restriction only (7.7 kg vs. 4.6 kg at 16 weeks; 5.2 kg vs. 1.0 kg at 1 year).

Table 1 presents an algorithm for determining a calorie and fat goal for patients in a weight-loss program.

Self-monitoring food intake is a key ingredient in teaching patients how to change their dietary intake. In our program, we encourage patients to write down all their food and the calories and grams of fat in each item; these records are kept every day for the first 6 months of treatment and then for at least 1 week each month. Subjects who are most successful at long-term weight control report that they have continued to self-monitor their intake.

Self-monitoring teaches patients a great deal about food. They learn what foods contribute most to their overall calorie and fat in-

T A B L E 1. *Setting a Calorie and Fat Goal for a Patient*

	Example
1. Estimate patient's current intake by multiplying current weight (in pounds) by 12	200 lb. × 12
Estimated Current Intake =	2,400 calories/day
2. To produce a 1- to 2-pound/week weight loss, prescribe a calorie goal that is 1,000 kcal lower than current intake	2,400 − 1,000
Prescribed Calorie Goal =	1,400 calories/day
3. Determine number of calories from fat for 20% fat intake	1,400 × .20
Calories From Fat =	280 calories/day
4. Divide calories from fat by 9 to determine number of fat grams to prescribe	280 ÷ 9
Prescribed Fat Goal =	31 g of fat/day

take and how to substitute low-calorie/low-fat foods. Self-monitoring also helps the patient and provider identify problem areas requiring further attention (e.g., high-calorie desserts, binge-eating episodes).

Another approach to help patients learn to make appropriate food choices is to provide patients with structured menus, indicating exactly what to eat at each meal, and grocery lists, indicating exactly what to purchase. Yet another approach is to provide the actual food for them to eat, in appropriate portion sizes, during the initial phase of the treatment. Recent studies have shown that food provisioning increases weight loss. These strategies also teach subjects more about the number of calories in food and improve the quality of the diet consumed.

CONSIDER VERY-LOW-CALORIE DIETS

Very-low-calorie diets (VLCDs) are diets of less than 800 kcal/day, usually prescribed as liquid formula or lean meat, fish, and fowl. These diets have been shown to be safe when used with carefully selected patients and appropriate medical monitoring. Advantages of these diets are as follows:

1. They produce fast initial weight losses, averaging 20 kg in 12 weeks. These initial weight losses can be very motivating to patients.
2. Patients with type II diabetes experience marked improvements in glycemic control within a few days of starting a VLCD. Approximately 50% of the overall improvement in glycemic control produced by losing 13 kg will occur within the first week of starting an 800 kcal diet.
3. Patients on VLCDs quickly recognize the relation between their eating and their glycemic control.

The major disadvantage of VLCDs is that they do not improve the magnitude of weight loss that is maintained long term. Subjects on VLCDs lose more weight initially, but then regain more weight than subjects on balanced low-calorie regimens. It remains unclear whether VLCDs promote better long-term glycemic control. If you choose to use VLCDs, keep this in mind and try to aggressively promote long-term maintenance of weight loss.

KEEP IN CONTACT WITH PATIENTS

Behavioral treatment programs developed in the 1970s usually lasted 10 weeks, and the weight losses achieved averaged 10 pounds. More recently, programs have been increased to 20 to 24 weeks, and weight losses approximate 20 pounds. Some researchers have used longer programs, with weekly meetings for a full year. Although such programs increase overall weight loss, subjects do not maintain a weight loss of 1 pound/week, so the cost-effectiveness of lengthening programs beyond 24 weeks becomes increasingly poor. Given this, the current approach is usually to begin treatment with 5 to 6 months of weekly group treatment.

After 20 to 24 weeks of intensive contact, it is important to continue to provide some type of contact for patients. Studies have shown that biweekly/weekly meetings involving therapist contact, aerobic exercise, and social support help patients maintain their weight loss. Contact by phone or mail has also been shown to be helpful.

IMPLEMENT BEHAVIOR MODIFICATION

It is often said that weight control programs should include diet, exercise, and behavior modification. However, behavior modification is not so much a separate component of a weight-loss program as it is a way of understanding and helping patients change their eating and exercise behaviors.

Behavior modification is based on the assumption that behaviors, such as eating and exercise, are learned. Thus, patients can learn new behaviors. Second, it is assumed that behaviors are controlled by the environment: both by 1) cues in the environment (such as the sight and smell of food) that set the stage for the behavior and by 2) reinforcers that come after the behavior and lead to its recurrence. Thus, to change behavior, it is important to change the environment that controls it. Key behavioral strategies (see Chapter 7) include self-monitoring to make patients aware of their behaviors; stimulus control techniques and preplanning to help patients change the environment they live in; and self-reinforcement and feedback to provide patients with reinforcement for their new behaviors.

CONCLUSION

A key component of all the strategies suggested above is to start slowly and allow the patient to experience initial success. This success will increase the patient's confidence that he or she can indeed lose weight.

ACKNOWLEDGMENTS

Preparation of this manuscript was supported by National Institutes of Health Grants DK-29757, HL-41330, and DK-46204.

BIBLIOGRAPHY

Jeffery RW, Wing RR, Thorson C, Burton LR, Raether C, Harvey J, Mullen M: Strengthening behavioral interventions for weight loss: a randomized trial of food provision and monetary incentives. *J Consult Clin Psychol* 61:1038–1045, 1993

National Task Force on the Prevention and Treatment of Obesity: Very low-calorie diets. *J Am Med Assoc* 270:967–974, 1993

Pascale RW, Wing RR, Butler BA, Mullen M, Bononi P: Effects of a behavioral weight loss program stressing calorie restriction versus calorie plus fat restriction in obese individuals with type II diabetes or a family history of diabetes. *Diabetes Care* 18:1241–1248, 1995

Perri MG, McAllister DA, Gange JJ, Jordan RC, McAdoo WG, Nezu AM: Effects of four maintenance programs on the long-term management of obesity. *J Consult Clin Psychol* 56:529–534,1988

Pronk NP, Wing RR: Physical activity and long-term maintenance of weight loss. *Obesity Res* 2:587–599, 1994

Wing RR, Koeske R, Epstein LH, Nowalk MP, Gooding W, Becker D: Long-term effects of modest weight loss in type II diabetic patients. *Arch Intern Med* 147:1749–1753, 1987

Smoking Cessation in Diabetes | 13

Edwin B. Fisher, Jr, PhD,
Sheryl L. Ziff, MA, and Debra
Haire-Joshu, PhD, RN

INTRODUCTION

Smoking is the greatest source of preventable death in our society, killing over 400,000 people each year, about 1 of every 6 or 7 deaths. More people die from heart disease related to smoking than from smoking-related cancers—a major reason smoking is a problem in diabetes. Cardiovascular risks of both smoking and diabetes are as high as 14 times those of either smoking or diabetes alone. Smoking is also associated with a heightened incidence of other diabetic complications, including retinopathy, neuropathy, and arterial occlusive disease. Nevertheless, the prevalence of smoking among diabetic adults may be even higher than in the population at large, 36 vs. 27% in one study. And the rate of smoking *cessation* appears to be lower among those with diabetes, 1 vs. 3 to 5% per year. For whatever reasons, smokers with diabetes are not getting the message. This chapter provides guidelines for smoking cessation in diabetes care.

GUIDELINES

Communicate the Importance of Smoking Cessation in Diabetes Care

Even if a clinician has addressed smoking, the message is not salient if said once, infrequently repeated, or delivered as something that "almost goes without saying" amidst other complex messages about diabetes care. Communicate the *priority* of smoking cessation with patients.

Because "everyone knows that smoking causes cancer," health professionals may think they don't need to remind patients of smoking's risks. But not everyone recognizes how many diseases are linked to smoking. And they don't recognize its impact on life expectancy—6 to 8 years on *average*—an impact that dwarfs that of other lifestyle risk factors.

When underestimating smoking's dangers is combined with a focus on the risks of diabetes, those with diabetes may discount smoking, "If I've got diabetes, I don't need to worry about lung cancer, so I may as well smoke." But, the synergistic risks for heart disease of both diabetes and smoking makes the combination especially lethal.

Communicate an Understanding of the Difficulty of Quitting Smoking

Several failed attempts usually precede successful cessation. Thus, smoking is a chronic problem, like diabetes, that needs to be treated chronically. Promote cessation with recognition that quitting is difficult and with understanding that the patient's failure to quit is not a sign of lack of concern or interest (see Table 1).

Emphasize the Clinician's Role as Key Authority and Catalyst

Many clinicians are frustrated with efforts to encourage smoking cessation and see themselves as unable to have much influence in this area. Although no single smoking intervention is highly successful, half of all adult smokers have quit. It is the combination of the clinician's efforts along with stop-smoking programs (such as those of the

TABLE 1. *Why Smoking Cessation Is Difficult*

◆ Nicotine is addictive. Cigarettes are an ideal vehicle for nicotine delivery. It takes approximately 7 seconds from inhalation for nicotine to reach the brain.

◆ Smoking is also conditioned. Cues in almost every setting and mood of daily life come to trigger urges to smoke.

◆ Addiction and conditioning intensify each other—association with numerous cues in daily life makes quitting nicotine more difficult. Being associated with a strong addictive drug makes the cues powerful triggers in almost every setting of daily life and makes quitting very hard.

◆ Advertising intensifies cigarettes as a symbol of success and independence, social and sexual attractiveness, or group identity, playing off many of the emotional effects of nicotine. Dollar for dollar of gross sales, cigarettes are three to four times as profitable as other consumer products. Thus, the would-be ex-smoker faces numerous relapse triggers in cigarette advertising.

From Fisher EB Jr, Lichtenstein E, Haire-Joshu D: Multiple determinants of tobacco use and cessation. In *Nicotine Addiction: Principles and Management.* Orleans CT, Slade JD, Eds. New York, Oxford University Press, 1993.

American Lung Association, the American Heart Association, and the American Cancer Society), educational campaigns, and increased government and private sector regulations that gets smokers to quit. Among these, the clinician's role has three crucial characteristics:

1. **Authority.** Patients with diabetes are especially likely to check with a diabetes care team before pursuing changes in health practices. Even a brief mention of smoking cessation may be helpful—but failure to mention it will also be heard.
2. **Access.** Most adults see a health provider at least once a year. This is especially likely for those with diabetes, who often receive medical care more than once a year.
3. **Catalyst.** The authority and access put health providers in a position to validate, potentiate, or catalyze the effects of all the other influences that encourage nonsmoking. Thus, even though a clinician's individual efforts may not have a high chance of success with each patient, the ability to catalyze and contribute to the aggregate of other nonsmoking influences is considerable.

TABLE 2. *Brief Counseling (3 minutes)*

- ◆ Inquire as to the patient's thoughts about quitting.

- ◆ Emphasize the importance of quitting in diabetes care.

- ◆ Encourage the patient to set quit date, make specific plans for coping with relapse triggers, and discuss with family and friends how they can add their cooperation or support.

- ◆ Refer the patient to a self-help or group cessation program for more extended counseling by other staff and/or for nicotine replacement.

Counsel All Patients Who Smoke to Quit

Simple, brief advice has been shown to increase significantly the likelihood of patients quitting. This counseling can be divided among the treatment team. Table 2 contains a brief counseling protocol and Table 3 a more extensive one.

Consider Nicotine Replacement

Nicotine replacement allows patients to split quitting into two tasks: 1) getting accustomed to life without all the smoking habits they have developed and 2) giving up nicotine altogether. But, nicotine replacement is an adjunct, not a magic bullet or a substitute for the patient's efforts to quit. It will not make anyone give up smoking. And, it does not remove the need for ongoing attention to and support for cessation efforts (see Table 4).

Smoking concurrent with patch use may cause an acute dangerous rise in blood nicotine levels. This rise is of special concern in those with cardiovascular disease. Firmly counsel patients to use the patch only when they have quit and to remove it if they resume any smoking.

Address Weight Gain

Smokers weigh less than nonsmokers, and quitters gain an average of 5 to 10 pounds. Emphasis on weight maintenance causes those with diabetes to fear weight gain following smoking cessation. Those with diabetes may also think that the risks of a 10-pound weight gain are

T A B L E 3. *Five- to Ten-Minute Counseling for Smoking Cessation*

1. Ask patients about their smoking status

- Have you ever smoked?
- Do you smoke now?
- What are your concerns or expectations about quitting?
- Have you thought about quitting?
- In the next 6 months?
- In the next month?
- Have you recently quit?

2. For those who have not thought about quitting

- Provide individualized information on the hazards of smoking.
- Emphasize increased risks of heart disease and diabetes complications arising from the combination of smoking and diabetes.
- Review benefits of smoking cessation: risks of heart disease, especially sudden death, decline within hours of cessation.
- Assure patients of willingness to assist in their efforts to quit and to review their thoughts about it the next time they come in.

3. For those thinking about quitting but not ready to quit (i.e., not in the next month)

- Review risks related to diabetes, etc., as above.
- Emphasize that benefits of quitting clearly outweigh difficulty and costs, especially in terms of heart disease, which is of special importance for those with diabetes.
- Point out the range of resources for smoking cessation, and help the patient access those resources.
- Express confidence in the patient's ability to quit.
- Discuss potential barriers to quitting (e.g., history of relapse, fear of weight gain).

4. For those about to quit or planning on quitting (e.g., in the next month)

- Review major steps of smoking cessation so that the patient can begin thinking about them:
  1. Setting a quit date appropriate to nature of habit (i.e., on a weekend if smoking is triggered by work stress).
  2. Identifying likely relapse triggers and making *specific* plans for coping with them *before* quitting.
  3. Recruiting cooperation and encouragement from family and friends.
- Assess for and discuss possibility of nicotine replacement.
- Discuss concerns about weight gain and other concerns related to diabetes and how they may be dealt with.
- Encourage the patient to talk with diabetes team or referral resources when ready to make a concrete plan.
- Make referral, prescribe nicotine replacement, provide self-help materials, or otherwise assist in specific plan.

Continued on next page

TABLE 3. *Continued*

---

5. At time of quit

♦ Help patient make plans to recruit support from family and friends.
♦ Arrange for support and monitoring by phone or clinic visit with team members.
♦ Review specific plans for coping with potential relapse triggers.

6. If patient has quit for at least 1 week

♦ Praise efforts, even if not flawless.
♦ Encourage vigilance; greatest threat to maintenance may be myth that, "I'm over the hump, feel pretty good, so I probably can have just a few (at parties, poker games, restaurants, on Wednesday nights, etc.)."
♦ Review strategies for avoiding triggers; encourage their continuance; better to err on the side of caution than recklessness.
♦ Review plan for support by family/friends or health-care team. Provide for team monitoring and encouragement if patient has little other access to these.
♦ Continue to discuss smoking and encourage vigilance regarding relapse for at least 6 months, preferably 1 year.

7. For those who have been ex-smokers for at least 1 year

♦ Note importance of continued nonsmoking.
♦ Express an eagerness to help if lapses occur.
♦ Reinforce success in smoking cessation to maintain it, to reflect its importance, and to build patient confidence for other aspects of diabetes management.

TABLE 4. *Guidelines for Nicotine Replacement*

Indicators: Smokes within 30 minutes of rising and/or at least one pack per day.

Timing: Use only following cessation of *all* smoking. The date of the prescription should reflect the patient's actual quit date so that commencement of patch therapy marks patient's initiating cessation. Discourage premature removal; research indicates insufficient dose and duration likely basis for relapse.

Concurrent Treatment: Encourage use of smoking cessation group, other support groups, or self-help materials. Follow up to assess patient response, including side effects as per package insert.

---

equivalent to those of smoking; in reality, the risk of smoking far out-weighs the risk of modest weight gain, even for those with diabetes.

When encouraging smoking cessation, be sure to acknowledge that very few patients will be able to quit smoking at the same time as focusing on weight management. Patients may not know that smoking cessation is important, even relative to the 5- to 10-pound weight gain to which it may lead. It may be helpful to acknowledge that previous emphasis on weight in diabetes care may have drawn attention away from the importance of smoking cessation. Reassure patients that once nonsmoking status is secure, they can work out a plan for losing the gained weight.

While emphasis on weight loss is relaxed, continue to encourage exercise and healthy eating. Exercise can provide substitute activity to distract the quitter from urges to smoke.

It is not clear when to return to a focus on weight management. The rate of relapse to smoking is especially high through most of the first 6 months after quitting, but levels off between 6 and 12 months. A guideline that is helpful is not to try to limit eating until the patient can do so without any noticeable return of desire for cigarettes. Otherwise, the patient is liable to stay on a merry-go-round of quitting smoking, gaining weight, returning to smoking to lose the weight, quitting smoking, gaining weight....

Refer Patients for Available Care

The American Lung Association, the American Heart Association, and the American Cancer Society provide materials for smoking cessation. Local chapters and many hospitals provide group smoking cessation classes and will be happy to supply materials for patients and arrange referral procedures.

Hypnosis is often considered as a resource. When used by bona fide professionals, hypnosis may contribute to smoking cessation efforts. However, when pursued as a "magic pill," it is unlikely to be successful.

If the patient has been treated for mood disturbance, the individual providing that care might be consulted with reference to the smoking cessation. Or, if the patient relies heavily on smoking to manage mood, referral for counseling may be helpful. If possible, have this counseling provided by someone with experience in smoking cessation.

Encourage Maintenance of Cessation

Cessation symptoms include acute cravings, irritability, lethargy (or increased energy), difficulty concentrating, headache, and changes in blood glucose. Reassure patients that these will pass within 3 to 10 days. Provide practical tips for combating these symptoms, but be aware that such tips may seem frivolous or common sense. These kinds of tips aren't really worthless, but they do need to match the individual. What's silly for one person may be a lifesaver for another. Instead of giving simple advice such as "take a nap," it may be better to encourage patients to use their own common sense and reassure them that their withdrawal symptoms are normal and not a sign of impending failure.

After the first week or so, patients will be over the worst of their withdrawal symptoms, but the process may become tedious. Paradoxically, patients' own success may trigger a feeling that they can have an occasional cigarette without returning to regular smoking. Long-term quitters frequently say that the most important thing they learned from their earlier failures was that they could not have "just one," and that, in the long run, it is easier simply to abstain than to try to control the addiction.

Frequent causes of relapse include environmental triggers (social situations, habitual smoking cues, pressure from peers), psychological triggers (negative moods, stress, flagging motivation to remain abstinent), and physiological cravings or withdrawal symptoms. Self-management strategies may minimize relapse triggers (see Table 5).

Address Relapse Paradox

Those who slip or relapse in the first weeks after quitting are far less likely to remain abstinent. It is important to encourage a clear determination not even to have "just one." On the other hand, it is also important to reinforce the patient's efforts if a lapse does occur and to

TABLE 5. *Essentials of Self-Management Strategies*

1. Identify details of the trigger situation. Good self-management strategies will vary according to the situation. For example, identify that the trigger is "telephone conversations with clients," not just "on the phone."

2a. Identify strategies to AVOID triggers before they gain control (e.g., go for a walk rather than sit at the far end of the table away from smokers during a coffee break).

OR

2b. Identify strategies to RESTRICT choices to smoke (e.g., go to a restaurant that doesn't allow smoking, so that after-dinner coffee and a cigarette won't be such a temptation).

3. Use relaxation procedures (tapes, meditation, muscle tension/release exercises, etc.) to prevent anxiety or stress from reaching levels likely to prompt relapse.

encourage resumption of the quit attempt. Many who have had relapses have gone on to success. It can be effective to explain this paradox to the patient in just these terms.

Patients may attribute their lapses to the task being impossible for them, to their own inability to succeed at it, to their being "just too addicted," or to other factors that are unchangeable and justify giving up the effort. Remind them that most long-term quitters have failed two to three times before succeeding. Encourage patients who have lapsed to review the details of the lapse situation and identify specific things they want to do differently the next time.

Address Emotional Factors Related to Diabetes

Smoking reduces anxiety and elevates mood. This makes it especially useful for those dealing with the stressors of diabetes. Additionally, smokers with diabetes report reluctance to give up the pleasures of smoking amidst all the other pleasures they see themselves as giving up because of their diabetes. For many patients, the encouragement and support of family, friends, and professionals will be especially important. Follow-up phone calls or patient visits may be helpful.

If periods of anxiety, low mood, or frustration are identified, teach patients to cope with these emotions as they would other potential triggers. The self-management strategies noted in Table 5 can be used to develop specific strategies for keeping moods from upsetting the cessation effort.

Arrange Varied and Ongoing Support

Follow up with a visit or phone call several days after the quit date, and then make several more contacts during the first several weeks. After this, titrate contacts from biweekly to monthly to bimonthly, but continue contacts for at least 6 months. In a comprehensive review of cessation studies in 1988, Kottke et al. concluded that "success was...the product of personalized smoking cessation advice and assistance, repeated in different forms by several sources over the longest feasible period." Since it is the variety and repetition of contact that are important, not any single key ingredient, staff can develop procedures for this that suit the practice setting and their own strengths.

Organize the Office Staff and Environment to Reflect the Importance of Smoking Cessation

One way to emphasize smoking cessation at the office is to appoint a member of the health-care team as a smoking cessation specialist. This person could provide more intensive counseling for cessation, perhaps coordinate secretarial staff in helping with follow-up contacts, and maintain supplies of self-help or other materials. Posters, clear signage prohibiting smoking, and pamphlets on smoking cessation make the clinic environment one that communicates the importance of non-smoking.

Patients must also be clear that the person who coordinates their care strongly endorses smoking cessation. That person should monitor and express interest in patients' progress. The risks of smoking and the well-documented effects of such clinical monitoring make any less attention to smoking cessation substandard practice.

Contribute to the Overall Campaign to Promote Nonsmoking

Assist and link up with public health, community, and mass media campaigns that encourage smoking cessation. For instance, an American Diabetes Association affiliate might cosponsor a program on smoking cessation on a local TV news channel and encourage individuals with diabetes to organize their own quit efforts around the television program. Or, an affiliate might promote locally available smoking cessation resources to its membership. Smoking cessation is accomplished not through any single strategy but through a combination of multiple strategies. Providers who assist in such broader activities can contribute to their patients' success.

BIBLIOGRAPHY

Fisher EB Jr, Lichtenstein E, Haire-Joshu D: Multiple determinants of tobacco use and cessation. In *Nicotine Addiction: Principles and Management.* Orleans CT, Slade JD, Eds. New York, Oxford University Press, 1993

Fisher EB Jr, Lichtenstein E, Haire-Joshu D, Morgan GD, Rehberg HR: Methods, successes, and failures of smoking cessation programs. In *Annual Review of Medicine.* Palo Alto, Annual Reviews, Inc., 1993, p. 481–513

Ford ES, Newman J: Smoking and diabetes mellitus: findings from 1988 behavioral risk factor surveillance system. *Diabetes Care* 14:871–874, 1991

Haire-Joshu D: Smoking cessation: a priority in diabetes care. *Diabetes Spectrum* 3:81–115, 1990

Haire-Joshu D: Smoking, cessation, and the Diabetes Health Care Team. *The Diabetes Educator* 17:54–67, 1991

Kottke TE, Battista RN, DeFriese GH: Attributes of successful smoking cessation interventions in medical practice: a meta-analysis of 39 controlled trials. *J Am Med Assoc* 259:2882–2889, 1988

United States Department of Health and Human Services: *How to Help Your Patients Stop Smoking: A National Cancer Institute Manual for Physicians.* Washington, DC, U.S. Govt. Printing Office, 1990 (NIH publ. no. 90-3064)

Preventing Eating Disorders in Young Women With Type I Diabetes

14

Wendy Satin Rapaport, PsyD,
Annette M. LaGreca, PhD, and
Paula Levine, PhD

INTRODUCTION

Weight concerns, body dissatisfaction, and dieting are common preoccupations among today's young women, so much so that it is often difficult to distinguish normal concerns about weight and dieting from more disturbed perceptions and eating patterns. The idea of an eating continuum with normal at one end, clinically diagnosed eating disorders at the other end, and subclinical aspects at varying points in between may be a useful way to view this problem.

Eating disorders can take a variety of forms. Bulimia nervosa is characterized by frequent episodes of binge eating that are accompanied by efforts to purge calories (e.g., self-induced vomiting, use of laxatives), as well as feelings of guilt and excessive concern about body image. Anorexia nervosa, on the other hand, is typically marked by severe restriction of caloric intake to the point where the individual is emaciated. This eating pattern is usually accompanied by fear of gaining weight and a distorted body image (i.e., the person feels fat even though emaciated). Both of these types of eating disorders have been found to occur in young women with diabetes, and they are associated with serious problems in glucose control as well as diabetic complications.

Although research does not clearly document a greater prevalence of clinical eating disorders in the diabetic population, approximately 1/3 of women taking insulin struggle with subclinical symptoms of eating disturbances, such as a preoccupation with thinness and self-image, feelings of guilt after eating certain foods, excessive exercise, binge eating, restrictive dieting, and misuse of insulin for weight control (i.e., omitting insulin to prevent weight gain similar to purging calories by vomiting, laxatives, or other methods). Unfortunately, individuals with even subclinical levels of eating disorders are at a markedly greater risk for developing complications from diabetes, such as neuropathy. Depression is also a serious concern in these young women.

Furthermore, research suggests that eating disorders are increasing in prevalence, are occurring at earlier ages, and are very resistant to treatment. Thus, it is critical for health-care professionals to become involved in the primary prevention of eating disorders. By educating and informing patients and their families, many eating disorders can be prevented from developing in the first place. This may be accomplished by emphasizing positive attitudes, feelings, and behaviors toward eating and diabetes care. Providers also need to examine their own biases about weight and body image, as they may unknowingly be communicated to patients. Secondary prevention, in the form of detecting the early warning signs of eating disorders, will also be an important goal for health-care providers. With these concerns in mind, this chapter focuses on some of the early warning signs of eating disorders, as well as strategies that health-care providers can use to help prevent disordered eating in their patients.

EARLY WARNING SIGNS OF EATING PROBLEMS

It is often difficult to detect clinical or subclinical eating disorders among patients with diabetes. Some potential markers for the development of an eating disorder in diabetes are listed below. If the patient has one or more of these markers, he or she may be struggling with an eating disorder. These markers are especially of concern among young women, who experience substantial social pressure to be "thin and beautiful" in our contemporary culture.

1. **Frequent diabetic ketoacidosis.** Frequent diabetic ketoacidosis (DKA) may be caused by omission of insulin. Many patients with serious eating disorders figure out how to avoid DKA that requires hospitalization to escape detection by family or clinicians; however, these patients do have elevated glycohemoglobin levels.

2. **Elevated hemoglobin A_{1c}.** Elevated hemoglobin A_{1c}, especially in a knowledgeable patient, may indicate the omission or reduction of insulin (i.e., insulin purging) to control weight or to avoid weight gain associated with binge eating.

3. **Anxiety about—or avoidance of—being weighed.** Anxiety about being weighed is often an indication of a negative body image, or of concern about potential criticism for being "overweight."

4. **Frequent and severe hypoglycemia.** Frequent and severe hypoglycemia could suggest an avoidance of eating and may otherwise result in a normal HbA_{1c}, thereby avoiding detection by family or medical providers.

5. **Nonadherence.** Nonadherence on most or all aspects of the diabetes regimen as reported by family members.

6. **Brittle diabetes.** Self-reports of extreme fluctuations in blood glucose.

7. **Delay in puberty or sexual maturation or failure to grow.** Otherwise, the person has a normal HbA_{1c}.

8. **Bingeing with food or alcohol.**

9. **Severe stress in the family.** Although eating problems, especially subclinical ones, can occur in "normal" families, certain psychosocial problems put youngsters at high risk for eating disorders. For example, child abuse, sexual abuse, parental divorce, and eating disorders among other family members can put an individual at high risk.

STRATEGIES FOR PRIMARY PREVENTION

Address Drive for Thinness and Body Dissatisfaction

Serious eating problems often develop during early adolescence. Research suggests that 50% of girls in the late elementary school years are already concerned about weighing too much. Given typical adolescent concerns about weight and body image, especially for girls, consider not emphasizing patients' weight or weight-loss goals. Discuss topics of heredity and "set point" contributing to body weight. Often there is a rapid weight loss before diagnosis of type I diabetes and then, with the initiation of insulin therapy, a rapid weight gain. If there has been substantial weight loss, help the patient regain the weight slowly in order to have time to adjust emotionally to the body changes. Prepare patients for temporary weight gain; if there is a weight gain, work closely with the patient to help normalize body image. Educate the patient about the politics of eating disorders; the ideal model-like shape is just not available to 99% of the women in the world, and the pursuit of thinness can interfere with success, popularity, happiness, and romance.

De-emphasize Diet and Dieting

The advent of a chronic disease that leads to considerable weight fluctuations and an intense (yet functional) focus on food can also create the right "climate" for an eating disorder. The American Diabetes Association's nutritional guidelines, updated in 1994, dramatically shifted views of healthy eating, emphasizing flexibility, choice, problem-solving, and individualization by age and tastes. This wording (e.g., flexibility versus forbidden, guidelines versus rules) is consistent with adolescent tasks of gaining mastery, control, and independence. The ADA guidelines stress eating in a healthy manner, the same as anyone. The guidelines talk about lifestyle and making gradual changes in eating habits. Families and health-care providers must not talk about diets, but rather about sensible eating.

Counsel Patients About the Need for Control and Expression of Negative Feelings About Diabetes Management

Even when diabetes onset precedes the teenage years, adolescence is associated with a deterioration of treatment adherence and metabolic control. Because of this, it is important that health-care providers allow for the expression of adolescents' irritation, frustration, and anger over their diabetes management and control, rather than dismissing these feelings as signs of moodiness, hormones, or blood glucose fluctuations.

It is important for health-care providers to appreciate how diabetes affects the person's perception of the important events in her life—such as friendships, social and sexual life, potential to have children, and career goals. Eating disorders can begin as a coping mechanism, as a way of being in control of one's life and needs: "Food is what I can control." Unfortunately, it is a poor external solution to important internal problems.

Individuals who have difficulty expressing themselves may act out their feelings. They may feel that they can stay in control by bingeing (in order to keep the feelings in) and purging (to let feelings go), without ever recognizing and dealing with their actual feelings. Rather than trying to control the patient's eating, insulin, or other aspects of diabetes, parents and health-care providers can be supportive and involved by working together. For example, help the patient to plan ahead for a difficult time, and act as her consultant. This may give her the freedom to make choices and have control over food and insulin usage.

Help With Conflict Over Normal Developmental Struggles

In most families, conflict arises over the normal development struggles of adolescence—such as achieving personal independence and autonomy without losing the support and involvement of family members. The diagnosis of diabetes can also disturb the adolescent's sense of self-control and self-esteem and can hinder the natural separation process between parent and child. Trying to find personal meaning in the diagnosis (i.e., "why me?") while trying to develop a positive self-identity becomes a very challenging task.

A particular vulnerability during adolescence is the need to fit in, to be accepted by peers, and to not be different. Encourage teens to identify at least one close friend with whom they can discuss their diabetes, and who can also be helpful and supportive in other social contexts. Peer support groups also provide a great opportunity to relate intimately to peers and help adolescents feel normal and less self-absorbed. Peer groups can also be instrumental in improving body image by encouraging exercise or sports that promote respect for one's body.

When a person has diabetes, typical adolescent thoughts about the future can raise fears about living independently, being loved, or having children. Providers can explore these issues by asking patients, "What picture do you have of yourself at age 30?" This can help the provider determine if there are any fears about the future that need to be examined. With encouragement of strategies for effective self-care behaviors, these concerns can be lessened.

Teach patients to say what they like about themselves and how they are handling their diabetes. Avoiding secrecy, feeling effective, and lessening guilt can promote self-esteem. Help patients identify their emotions, overcome their cognitive distortions, and participate in open, honest exchanges.

Address Metabolic Reactivity

Further complicating this developmental period, and potentially contributing to eating disorders, are the frequent metabolic fluctuations that accompany diabetes during adolescence. These can take the form of weight changes and of physical feelings associated with high and low blood glucose (e.g., fatigue, irritability). The typical adolescent self-absorption and fixation with body image is magnified by diabetes.

Blood glucose changes affect mood changes that are already occurring in adolescence. Distinguish compliance from control: "I followed the rules (my behavior was OK), but my blood sugar didn't." Metabolic control is not a moral issue or self-esteem rating. Encourage openness about glucose readings. Also, remind patients that adherence, especially during adolescence, may not lead to positive outcomes (e.g., hormonal changes→insulin resistance). Parents must be reminded of this, so they can avoid being judgmental and can reinforce their youngster's honesty. Health-care providers may need to practice becoming comfortable saying, "I'm glad you're telling me you haven't been testing."

Recognize and treat depression with therapy (refer to mental health specialists) and medication (psychiatry). Also, recognize that stress, as well as hormonal changes, may elicit eating as a coping mechanism.

Involve the Family

Especially for the newly diagnosed, elicit feelings of all family members (fathers and siblings are often neglected) concerning turmoil and family conflict about diabetes; help guide the grief process rather than covering it up. Help the young patient to grieve *consciously*, so that he or she will not become disconnected from feelings about diabetes and redirect grief to body image. Consider support groups as a formal vehicle for grief.

Identify the normal, *acute* grieving process to avoid a *chronic* pathological response. Allow the healthy expression of sadness and anger to have a voice rather than be submerged and acted out on issues of thin, fat, or food. Redefine the "good patient" as one who expresses annoyance, resentment, embarrassment, etc.

Family management of diabetes requires openness, organization, and positive coping skills. Excessive concerns prior to diagnosis regarding body image, food, weight, perfectionism, achievement, or approval put patients at risk. Early intervention with the whole family is crucial. Diabetes is not a short-term crisis; it's an ongoing situation that must be managed.

Facilitate Empowerment

Try to give patients unconditional positive regard and avoid encouraging patients to please or to rebel through poor diabetic control. Be happy to see patients regardless of their weight, monitoring, or blood glucose results. Encourage self-expression and self-evaluation by using an empowerment model (see Chapter 17):

> "Tell me what it feels like to go low and have to eat when you're trying to diet. What goes through your mind? What do you feel like doing?"

> Be careful not to say:
> "Your blood sugars are great!"
> "You're wonderful!"

"You never follow your meal plan."
"Don't you care about yourself?"

Judgments lead to self-worth being based on outcomes; self-esteem must not be based on what the person weighs or on their blood glucose levels. If a patient loses weight, be careful not to say, "You look wonderful, you've lost so much weight." Try instead, "It's wonderful to see you. How do you think things are going for you?"

CONCLUSION

Health-care professionals have an ideal opportunity to become actively involved in the primary prevention of eating disorders among youth with diabetes. This may be accomplished by practicing and using the strategies we have outlined above. In addition, prevention often involves identifying mental health specialists who are knowledgeable in diabetes, who can serve as consultants to the health-care team, and who may be direct referral sources for patients and families when there is an intense or prolonged problem. Health-care providers can provide a supportive context for patients and families, so that they can deal with emotional problems that arise. Teach patients to become critical thinkers, to develop successful coping strategies for dealing with the stress of diabetes, and to avoid associating body image or glucose control with success, intelligence, or achievement. This way of working with patients and their families may be difficult and time-consuming, at least initially, but in the long run it can also be very rewarding.

BIBLIOGRAPHY

Beck A: *Cognitive Therapy and the Emotional Disorders.* New York, International University Press, 1976

Fairburn CG, Peveler RC, Davies B, Mann JI, Mayor RA: Eating disorders in young adults with insulin-dependent diabetes mellitus. *Br Med J* 303:11–20, 1991

LaGreca AM, Auslander WF, Greco P, Spetter D, Fisher EB Jr, Santiago JV: I get by with a little help from my family and friends: adolescents' support for diabetes care. *J Pediatr Psychol* 20:449–476, 1995

LaGreca AM, Schwartz LT, Satin W: Eating patterns in young women with IDDM: another look. *Diabetes Care* 10:657–660, 1987

Marcus MD, Wing RR: Eating disorders and diabetes: diagnosis and management. *Diabetes Spectrum* 3:361–397, 1990

Rodin GM, Daneman D: Eating disorders and IDDM: a problematic association. *Diabetes Care* 15:1402–1412, 1992

Zerbe K: *The Body Betrayed: Women, Eating Disorders and Treatment* Washington, DC, American Psychiatric Press, 1993

Recognizing and Managing Depression in Patients With Diabetes

15

Patrick J. Lustman, PhD, Linda S. Griffith, MSW, and Ray E. Clouse, MD

INTRODUCTION

The term depression denotes two distinctly different experiences. The first is the common experience: occasional periods of feeling down, irritable, stressed, or just generally out-of-sorts. These depressed feelings are usually short-lived and inconsequential. A bad day is followed by a good day, and life goes on. The second is the experience of depression as a serious, sometimes life-threatening mental disorder. This depression is conferred the status of a medical diagnosis named major depressive disorder. The disorder presents as a cluster of mental (e.g., sadness, loss of interest) and physical (e.g., fatigue, sleep difficulties) symptoms that persist over an extended period of time and significantly impair interpersonal behavior, occupational functioning, and quality of life. In this chapter, the term depression is used as a synonym for this severe form of depression, major depressive disorder.

FREQUENCY, CAUSES, AND CONSEQUENCES OF DEPRESSION IN DIABETES

Approximately 5 to 8% of the general population will experience a major depressive disorder at some point during their lifetime. The disorder is roughly three times more prevalent in those with diabetes, affecting 15 to 20% of patients. Depression is equally common in patients with either type I or type II diabetes. Although a gender difference has not been proven, the available studies suggest that depression in those with diabetes occurs more frequently in women than men, much as it does in the general United States population. The fact that depression is more common in people with diabetes does not prove that diabetes causes depression or that depression causes diabetes. Prevalence findings alone do not establish cause-and-effect relationships. Perhaps most importantly, the frequent co-occurrence of depression and diabetes establishes that these conditions will have many opportunities to affect one another.

For the present, the cause of depression in people with diabetes is unknown, but probably is complex, resulting from an interaction among psychological, physical, and genetic factors. The precise contribution of these factors will vary from patient to patient. Diabetes is a demanding condition, and adjusting to dietary restrictions, treatment regimens, hospitalizations, and increased financial obligations can be difficult for patients and their loved ones. Coping with limitations in function associated with advancing diabetes, such as loss of vision or sexual capacity, is certainly stressful and may contribute to depression. Various physical changes associated with diabetes, including neurochemical and neurovascular abnormalities, also are factors. Lastly, there is information to suggest that depression in people with diabetes may be caused by genetic factors unrelated to diabetes. Each of these potential sources should be considered when speculating the cause of depression in any particular patient.

Whatever the cause, depression, once present, will interact negatively with diabetes. The pervasive nature of its adverse effects is striking. A model of the interactions is shown in Figure 1 and discussed below. A more extensive discussion of the causal nature of these relationships is available elsewhere (see Bibliography). Depression at the epicenter of the model intersects with every other box. It has been directly associated with poor glycemic control, the major cause of diabetes complications. Depression also contributes to obesity, physical inactivity, and treatment noncompliance, factors that promote poor glycemic control. Depression has been related directly to an increased risk of neuropathy and cardiovascular disease and to other factors (smoking and substance abuse) that add further to their risk. Thus, depression has direct and indirect links to both poor glycemic control

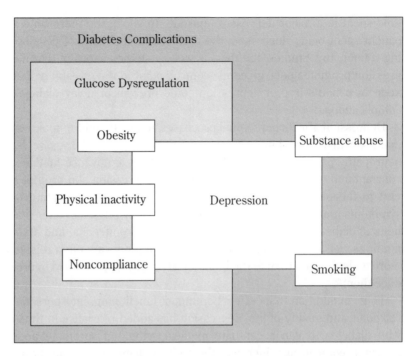

F I G U R E 1. Depression has been associated with many behavioral and medical factors in diabetic patients. Both depression and its associated factors have been linked to glucose dysregulation and diabetes complications. Intersecting boxes in this figure indicate significant associations proven in diabetes research. Adapted from Lustman PJ (Guest Editor): Depression in adults with diabetes. *Diabetes Spectrum* 7:161–189, 1994.

and diabetes complications. Finally, depressed patients respond poorly to lifestyle interventions (e.g., smoking cessation and weight-loss programs), further jeopardizing efforts to control diabetes and improve outcome.

Evidence linking depression to diabetes complications continues to accumulate. In a noteworthy recent study by Kovacs and colleagues, a group of children and adolescents underwent careful and repeated psychiatric and diabetes evaluations over the 10-year period following diagnosis of type I diabetes. The methods used made it possible to calculate precisely the amount of time subjects spent in depression and in poor glycemic control over this 10-year interval. The results showed that the risk of developing retinopathy was related to three factors: duration of type I diabetes, time spent in poor glycemic control, and time spent in a major depressive episode. In short, the more time a patient spent being depressed, the greater the likelihood of developing retinopathy. Studies like this, as well as studies showing that depression promotes poor glycemic control, point to the possibility that keeping patients free of depression could prevent or delay diabetes complications.

Depression affects perceptual processes and is thought to make us more sensitive to, and intolerant of, physical symptoms. For example, neuropathy pain that is normally an intermittent annoyance may feel constant and unbearable during a period of depression and prompt a visit to the physician. Depression even influences the reporting of symptoms that are usually considered exclusively physical manifestations of diabetes. Research has shown that gastrointestinal and autonomic as well as hyper- and hypoglycemic symptoms are often related more to depression than to the biomedical processes presumed to produce them.

Thus, in addition to its effects on mood, functioning, interpersonal relations, and quality of life, depression has added relevance in those with diabetes. It can accentuate medical symptoms, promote poor glycemic control, and increase the risk of diabetes complications. Because of these interactions, the clinical presentation of diabetes may actually suggest the presence of depression. Depression should be considered 1) when symptoms of hyper- or hypoglycemia persist in the face of objective evidence of adequate glycemic control, 2) when other symptoms lack a solid medical explanation or are out of proportion to the objective findings, 3) when sexual dysfunction is raised as a concern, or 4) whenever chronic pain is a dominant complaint.

IDENTIFICATION OF DEPRESSION IN DIABETES

Using currently accepted psychiatric diagnostic techniques, the diagnosis of major depressive disorder is made when a number of criterion symptoms occur together, are severe, and persist daily over a period of at least 2 weeks (Table 1). Sad mood or a significant loss of interest or pleasure are the *sine qua non* for the diagnosis, and one or the other must be present along with any four of the other listed symptoms. The symptoms must be the source of significant distress or decline in social, occupational, or other important areas of functioning in order to count toward a diagnosis of depression. Criterion

T A B L E   1. *Diagnostic Criteria for Major Depressive Disorder*

1. One of the following:
 ◆ Depressed mood
 ◆ Markedly diminished interest or pleasure in almost all activities

2. Four of the following:
 ◆ Significant weight loss or gain
 ◆ Insomnia or hypersomnia
 ◆ Psychomotor agitation or retardation
 ◆ Fatigue, loss of energy
 ◆ Feelings of worthlessness or guilt
 ◆ Impaired concentration or indecisiveness
 ◆ Recurrent thoughts of death or suicide

3. Symptoms must be present most of the day.

4. Symptoms must be present nearly daily for ≥2 weeks.

5. Symptoms must be the result of significant distress or impairment and not be attributable to medications, medical conditions, or bereavement.

All five criteria are required.

symptoms that result from taking medication or illicit drugs or that are referable to bereavement are discounted.

One additional rule must be considered in valuing these symptoms. Those judged as being caused by a medical condition do not help in establishing the diagnosis of depression. Because uncontrolled diabetes can cause some of the very symptoms typical of depression (e.g., fatigue, weight changes), the rule is useful and discourages overdiagnosis of the emotional disorder. The fact that diabetes does not directly produce the key diagnostic symptoms (sadness and loss of interest or pleasure) further reduces the likelihood of a false-positive diagnosis. In short, diabetes, even when uncontrolled, does not impair the clinician's ability to easily and accurately diagnose depression.

Despite its potential for diagnosis, depression in people with diabetes is recognized and treated in fewer than one-third of cases. Many factors contribute to this problem, including the assumption that depression is merely secondary to diabetes and not of independent importance. The perception persists despite clear evidence that depression may interact negatively with diabetes, and it unfortunately serves to focus clinical management efforts exclusively on the medical condition.

Depression in the medically ill also may go unrecognized because clinicians generally do not have the time and training required to perform formal psychodiagnostic interviews. Brief paper-and-pencil screening instruments capable of detecting depression can help with this problem. These instruments are well-suited to the realities of making psychiatric diagnoses in outpatient medical settings. For example, the 21-item Beck Depression Inventory (BDI) does not require an interview, is self-administered, takes 5 to 10 minutes to complete, and is scored easily and manually by summing the ratings for each of the 21 items.

We recommend that patients with depression symptoms lasting 2 weeks or more and BDI scores ≥16 undergo formal diagnostic testing to determine whether major depressive disorder is present. This cutoff score captures more than 70% of the patients with depression. In situations where resources are more plentiful and the emphasis is on not overlooking depression cases, the BDI cutoff score could be lowered to 12, a score that would capture at least 90% of patients with diagnosable depression.

COURSE AND MANAGEMENT OF DEPRESSION IN DIABETES

Depression in diabetes is a recurring condition in which periods of depression alternate with periods of feeling normal or well. Only about 20% of diabetic patients who recover from an episode of depression remain well for more than 5 years. Treatment of depression in patients with diabetes presumably would help them get better faster and remain well longer, but very little systematic information relevant to this presumption is available. Thus, the treatment recommendations that follow are blended from what is known about depression management in patients without a chronic medical illness and the little information available in patients with diabetes.

There are two general methods for treating depression: one is medication and the other is psychotherapy. Psychotherapy differs from general supportive counseling in its application of a specific set of proven techniques aimed at removing depression symptoms and improving psychosocial functioning. In general, medication and psychotherapy are equally effective treatments for depression, and approximately 50 to 60% of treated patients will achieve a remission within 3 months. There is evidence that some patients may benefit from the combination of medication and psychotherapy, but little information is available to guide the clinician in selecting patients for this approach. Initial treatment is often predetermined by the patient's selection of a mental health professional. Primary care physicians and diabetologists are most likely to treat depression with medication and common-sense advice. Psychologists and social workers employ counseling and formal psychotherapy. Psychiatrists may use a combination of these treatments but generally emphasize medication.

Consideration of the individual symptom picture provides a logical basis for effective treatment planning, because the depression "syndrome" usually includes symptoms in addition to those used in making the diagnosis of depression. For example, the first choice of treatment for depression dominated by somatic symptoms might be medication, whereas psychotherapy would be a well-chosen treatment for depression characterized by interpersonal difficulties. Psychotherapy is also the treatment of choice for patients who want to learn coping or self-management techniques aimed at removing depression and preventing its recurrence. Medication is more appropriate for patients who do not have the time or financial resources for psychotherapy or who are simply not inclined to talk about their problems. The presence of suicidal ideation requires access to the full range of depression treatments, and suicidal patients are most often referred to a psychiatrist. Additional thought must be given to the impact of treatment on the medical disease. For example, one class of antidepressant medications might be more desirable than another for a diabetic patient with heart disease or gastroparesis.

Antidepressant agents commonly used to treat depression along with their doses and side effects are shown in Table 2. These medications are equal in their antidepressant effects when used in primary care settings and psychiatric clinics, and the same is presumed in diabetic samples. Consequently, selection is based on such factors as presenting symptoms, coexisting medical conditions, drug interactions, and side effects. The conventional tricyclic antidepressants have been used effectively in primary care for more than 40 years and are particularly helpful in regulating sleep. Use of these agents in patients with diabetes must take into consideration the potential for weight gain, orthostatic hypotension, and other adverse cardiovascular effects. The newer selective serotonin reuptake inhibitors (SSRIs) are equally effective but do not usually cause weight gain or sedation. Their use in diabetes must be balanced against the possibility of gas-

TABLE 2. *Selected Antidepressant Medications, Dosage, and Side Effects*

Drug	Therapeutic Dosage Range (mg/day)	Side Effect						
		Anti-cholinergic	Central Nervous System		Cardiovascular		Other	
			Drowsiness	Insomia/Agitation	Orthostatic Hypotension	Cardiac Arrhythmia	Gastrointestinal Distress	Weight Gain (> 6 kg)
Tricyclics								
Amitriptyline	75–300	4	4	0	4	3	0	4
Desipramine	75–300	1	1	1	2	2	0	1
Imipramin	75–300	3	3	1	4	3	1	3
Nortriptyline	40–200	1	1	0	2	2	0	1
Heterocyclics								
Amoxapine	100–600	2	2	2	2	3	0	1
Bupropion	225–450	0	0	2	0	1	1	0
Trazodone	150–600	0	4	0	1	1	1	1
SSRIs								
Fluoxetine	10–40	0	0	2	0	0	3	0
Paroxetine	20–50	0	0	2	0	0	3	0
Sertraline	50–150	0	0	2	0	0	3	0

Adapted from U.S. Department of Health and Human Services, Agency for Health Care Policy and Research, Depression Guideline Panel: *Depression in Primary Care: Volume 2. Treatment of Major Depression* (Clinical Practice Guidelines, no. 5). Washington, DC, U.S. Government Printing Office (AHCPR publ. no. 93-0551), 1993. Relative occurrence of side effects among agents listed: ranked from 0 (absent or rare) to 4 (relatively common). Anticholinergic includes dry mouth, blurred vision, urinary hesitancy, and constipation.

trointestinal distress, agitation, and sexual dysfunction. The monoamine oxidase inhibitors and electroconvulsive therapy are usually considered only for severe depressions that do not respond to the treatments described above.

Psychotherapy may have a uniquely important role in the treatment of depression because it has no physical side effects contraindicating its use in diabetes. Cognitive therapy (CT) and interpersonal therapy (IPT) are psychotherapeutic treatments with proven antidepressant efficacy. CT evolved from observations that depressed people think in stereotypic ways ("I hate myself, my life stinks, and I have no future"). Depression is removed by teaching patients to identify, challenge, and replace these depressing thought patterns. IPT views depression as arising in an interpersonal context in which stressful and conflicted relationships are thought to cause, maintain, and exacerbate depression. Treatment involves the teaching of specific communication and social skills. This therapy may be particularly relevant in diabetes because changes in roles and functioning occur frequently as the medical disease worsens. Both CT and IPT teach skills that help patients better cope with stressful life circumstances and thus may be useful not only in removing depression but also in preventing its recurrence.

A multitude of logistic, financial, and personal issues may also affect choice of depression treatment. For example, what is the patient's preference for treatment? A therapeutic alliance and increased compliance is best established when patients are involved in the treatment process. Does age, physical mobility, or mental acuity restrict treatment options? Does the patient's employment or lifestyle allow time for treatment? What are the patient's resources in terms of money and access to medical and mental health professionals? In this era of managed care, out-of-pocket expenses can be considerable for the modestly insured patient.

CONCLUSION

Depression in people with diabetes is a prevalent and chronic condition. It has importance in diabetes that goes beyond its recognized effects on normal mental functioning. Depression will actually complicate the medical disease by influencing the reporting of diabetes symptoms, reducing compliance, promoting poor glycemic control, and increasing the risk of progressive end-organ damage. Brief paper-and-pencil tests like the Beck Depression Inventory can be used in outpatient medical settings to screen for depression and help focus the health-care team on patients in need of treatment. Treatment of depression is effective and important for its positive effects on mood, glycemic control, and overall quality of life.

ACKNOWLEDGMENTS

Preparation of this manuscript was supported by National Institutes of Health Grant DK-36452 and a Clinical Research Grant from the American Diabetes Association.

BIBLIOGRAPHY

American Psychiatric Association: *Diagnostic and Statistical Manual of Mental Disorders*. 4th ed. Washington, DC, American Psychiatric Association, 1994

Beck AT, Beamesderfer A: Assessment of depression: the depression inventory. *Mod Probl Pharmacopsychiatry* 7:151–169, 1974

Gavard JL, Lustman PJ, Clouse RE: Prevalence of depression in adults with diabetes: an epidemiological evaluation. *Diabetes Care* 16:1167–1178, 1993

Kovacs M, Mukerji P, Drash A, Iyengar S: Biomedical and psychiatric risk factors for retinopathy among children with IDDM. *Diabetes Care* 18:1592–1599, 1995

Lustman PJ (Guest Editor): Depression in adults with diabetes. *Diabetes Spectrum* 7:161–189, 1994

Lustman PJ, Griffith LS, Gavard JA, Clouse RE: Depression in adults with diabetes. *Diabetes Care* 15:1631–1639, 1992

U.S. Department of Health and Human Services, Agency for Health Care Policy and Research, Depression Guideline Panel: *Depression in Primary Care: Volume 2. Treatment of Major Depression* (Clinical Practice Guidelines, no. 5). Washington, DC, U.S. Government Printing Office (AHCPR publ. no. 93-0551), 1993

PREVENTION OF SPECIAL PROBLEMS IV

The chapters in this section address different facets of the patient-provider relationship.

In the first chapter, Rubin and Peyrot discuss patients' emotional functioning at diagnosis. Specific recommendations are given to help clinicians deal with and prevent the most common psychological struggles of newly diagnosed patients.

In the second chapter, R. Anderson, Funnell, and Arnold suggest the empowerment approach for helping patients change their self-care behaviors. Through examples of specific patients, we see how the clinician's use of the empowerment approach can help patients make progress toward healthy lifestyle choices that affect their diabetes control. The foundation of the empowerment approach is that human beings make and maintain behavior changes successfully if the changes are individually meaningful and individually chosen. This truth is woven through the chapters by Hanson and Polonsky that follow.

Hanson addresses the other side of the patient-provider relationship and explains what happens when diabetes clinicians burn out. Hanson's chapter provides a careful look at the factors that contribute to provider burnout, as well as practical strategies for preventing this problem for clinicians who care for patients with diabetes.

Polonsky's chapter continues with the theme of burnout, applying it to patients with diabetes. This chapter details how, as diabetes progresses, the frustrations of daily attention to a complex task like diabetes management can lead to an overwhelmed, overstressed state in many patients. Polonsky focuses on practical strategies for treating patients with diabetes burnout.

Emotional Responses to Diagnosis | 16

Richard R. Rubin, PhD, CDE, and
Mark Peyrot, PhD

INTRODUCTION

The period following diabetes onset and diagnosis can be a time of crisis for many people. Clinical and subclinical emotional difficulties may be triggered by this crisis, and existing emotional problems may be exacerbated. Emotional problems severe enough to warrant a psychiatric diagnosis—most often depression or anxiety disorder—are common in recently diagnosed children and are seen often in recently diagnosed adults, as well. It is important for clinicians to closely monitor emotional reactions to diagnosis in their patients so that appropriate treatment can be instituted early, when the benefits are greatest. Effective treatment can restore emotional equilibrium: a worthy goal in its own right. Moreover, it is equally important for clinicians to address dysfunctional emotional responses, because they may have a detrimental effect by inhibiting effective diabetes self-care. The goal of this chapter is to offer information and guidelines for treating emotional problems and disorders in individuals with newly diagnosed diabetes. Many of the issues addressed here may also apply to patients with diabetes of longer duration.

RECOGNIZE DENIAL WHEN IT IS PRESENT AT DIAGNOSIS

Denial is a common response to diagnosis, especially among patients with type II diabetes, since for them, diabetes onset is much less dramatic and the symptoms are often more subtle than those in type I diabetes. While most view denial as negative, we believe that this response is natural at diagnosis; the negative consequences that may follow from denial, and not denial per se, are the problem. Denial can even be healthy, if it protects newly diagnosed patients from becoming emotionally overwhelmed. Maintaining emotional equilibrium is essential for establishing effective self-care.

Denial is destructive when it makes effective management impossible. Destructive denial can be difficult to identify. The external appearance of not being concerned about diabetes and its management may result from two quite different emotional foundations. On the one hand, patients may be unaware of the seriousness of diabetes. On the other hand, patients may be extremely threatened by diabetes and may use denial as a way of coping with their fear.

Patients' emotional responses can be ascertained indirectly by asking about diabetes-related attitudes and perceptions. Factors that may contribute to intense fear include perception of a need for unmanageable changes in lifestyle or a family history of diabetes-related poor outcomes. Lack of concern may result from a belief that diabetes has few consequences or from misinformation, such as the belief that if one does not have to take insulin, the diabetes is not serious.

ADDRESS DENIAL DIRECTLY AND EFFECTIVELY

Avoid contributing to denial by "soft pedaling" the diagnosis, i.e., telling the patient that he or she has "borderline diabetes," "mild diabetes," or "a touch of sugar." This approach may lead the patient to believe that diabetes is not serious and effective management not important. The opposite approach, describing diabetes and its potential consequences in devastating terms, may also contribute to destructive denial, especially for a patient who is using denial to cope with excessive fear. Fear-inducing communication may lead the patient to feel hopeless and adopt an ostrich-like approach to diabetes and its management. Thus, clinicians may want to make sure they know which type of patient they are dealing with before choosing an information-giving strategy. Careful questioning, as described in Chapters 17 and 19, can be helpful in this regard.

To avoid destructive denial, newly diagnosed patients need accurate complete information, presented in stages and directed to meeting their specific needs and learning styles. If patients are using denial to cope with fear, help them focus on how it is possible to dramatically reduce their chances of having complications by effective self-care. If patients' denial arises from a lack of concern, make sure they are aware of the seriousness of diabetes and the potential negative consequences of ineffective self-care. Once the proper emotional context has been established, help patients develop self-care skills to enable them to effectively manage their diabetes. Specific barriers may be addressed through formal diabetes education, nutritional counseling, and coping skills training. Coping skills training refers to formal and informal efforts to address psychosocial barriers to effective self-care.

SCREEN FOR OTHER EMOTIONAL PROBLEMS

Another response to intense fear is catastrophizing or emphasizing the worst aspects of the disease; for example, that one will get all the complications of diabetes no matter what one does. This response looks very different from denial, although it may have some of the same emotional antecedents. Patients who exhibit this response often feel overwhelmed and have given up as far as their self-care, i.e., they suffer from diabetes burnout. For more on working with patients who suffer from diabetes burnout, see Chapter 19.

Anger is another emotion that may be seen at diagnosis. This anger may be based on the belief that diabetes represents an unfair and unbearable burden. Intense anger may preclude an effective approach to identifying the changes that are necessary in order to successfully live with diabetes.

Finally, sadness (or subclinical depression) is also common at diagnosis. Sadness may reflect a mourning process for a loss of health and freedom of lifestyle. Patients who emphasize the negative aspects of diabetes may lose the will to respond to the challenge of managing their disease.

INVOLVE THE FAMILY AND ENTIRE MEDICAL STAFF IN TREATING EMOTIONAL PROBLEMS

The painful emotions that often arise at diagnosis must be respected. Acknowledge these emotions and address them before attempting to teach diabetes management. Open-ended questions concerning diabetes-related feelings may help some patients recognize and acknowledge their emotions. The beliefs that underlie these emotions must also be addressed. Let the patient know that early adjustment to living with diabetes can be difficult. Take advantage of "teachable moments" (i.e., situations when motivation is high) to reinforce the patient's efforts to deal with the emotional and practical aspects of life with diabetes.

View the patient's family as an essential source of support. Include them whenever possible. Refer patients to support groups, offer recommendations for periodical literature, videotapes, pamphlets, and books that deal with the emotional side of diabetes. Finally, encourage patients to join the American Diabetes Association and other organizations whose activities may facilitate acceptance.

HELP PATIENTS BALANCE EFFECTIVE SELF-CARE WITH GOOD QUALITY OF LIFE

Some patients, especially those with type I diabetes who engage in intensive management, may respond to the anxiety they feel at diagnosis by obsessive preoccupation with tight control and compulsive efforts to achieve normoglycemia. This kind of behavior is the opposite of denial and may be thought of as too much of a good thing.

When encouraging patients to initiate effective self-care at diagnosis, be aware that this advice might fuel obsessive-compulsive tendencies in certain predisposed individuals.

It is often hard to draw the line between effective intensive management and an obsessive-compulsive approach, especially at the outset. These differences may be clearer in the months following diagnosis. The best indicator is the comfort the patient feels with the regimen, especially if the regimen is an intensive one. Once again, careful questioning is probably the best way to identify those whose approach to treatment is obsessive-compulsive. Useful questions include, "How much do you worry when your blood glucose goes high?" and "How strict are you about sticking to your regimen?"

Patients with obsessive-compulsive tendencies may say they have to be perfect: to eat *exactly* the same amount at *exactly* the same time every day, to do many blood glucose tests every day, and to stick precisely to the regimen even when it disrupts other aspects of life, such as social relations, work, and family life.

The issue of the patient's comfort with his or her behavior is the key to understanding the behavior. Some people stick closely to schedules for diabetes-related activities and significantly adjust other aspects of their lives, yet do this without feeling driven. Good self-care 1) focuses on the dual goals of maintaining good metabolic control and a fairly normal life, 2) is flexible in the pursuit of these goals, and 3) makes the diabetes regimen a matter-of-fact, albeit very important, part of life, not a painful preoccupation that negates all other aspects of living.

If a patient appears to be sacrificing quality of life for rigid regimen adherence, address the issue directly, emphasizing several guidelines for balancing the need to "do the right thing" with the equally important need to "live (fairly) normally." First, extremes are unworkable. Finding a personally acceptable balance is the key to success. Perfection is unattainable even with the most heroic efforts, and an unbending effort to achieve perfection is a recipe for eventual breakdown.

Second, with practice, each person can find workable approaches to most diabetes-related situations. This will seem difficult or impossible at first, but with support and counseling, solutions can be found.

SCREEN FOR DEPRESSION AND ANXIETY DISORDER

Clinical depression and anxiety can severely hamper medical management of diabetes. It is well recognized that feelings of hopelessness and helplessness often associated with depression may contribute to a disastrous negative cycle of poor self-care, worsened glycemia, and deepened depression. There are also recent suggestions that the symptoms of depression and hyperglycemia may exacerbate each other at a neuroendocrine level. In addition, there is evidence that the natural course of depression is more devastating in patients who have diabetes than it is in individuals who have no medical problems. In people with diabetes, depressive episodes may occur more frequently, be more severe, and last longer. For more on depression and diabetes, see Chapter 15.

Like depression, anxiety disorder may interfere with effective diabetes management. The state of anxiety interferes with learning diabetes self-management skills. Acute stress may trigger neuroendocrine responses leading to hyperglycemia. In addition, certain specific fears—refusal to take insulin or an overwhelming fear of ever becoming hypoglycemic, for instance—may represent significant barriers to effective management.

It is important to identify depression in newly diagnosed individuals when it is present and to provide effective treatment. Unfortunately, the task of diagnosing depression in patients with diabetes can be problematic because many of the most common symptoms of depression, including insomnia, fatigue, appetite disturbances, and decreased libido, are also symptoms of hyperglycemia. Since many people with diabetes are hyperglycemic at diagnosis, the presence of affective symptoms, such as guilt, anhedonia (markedly diminished interest or pleasure in almost all activities), and feelings of helplessness or worthlessness, memory impairment, and indecision, are particularly useful for an accurate diagnosis.

Some symptoms of anxiety disorder are similar to those of depression. These include fatigue, sleep disturbance, difficulty concentrating, and irritability. Other symptoms of anxiety disorder include restlessness and muscle tension. As with depression, some symptoms of anxiety disorder overlap with those of metabolic disregulation. In the case of anxiety disorder, these are symptoms of hypoglycemia.

For patients who may be depressed or anxious, ask direct questions concerning feelings of sadness, apathy, irritability, difficulty concentrating, fatigue, sleep disturbance, and a decreased capacity for pleasure. Screen patients for depression by assessing factors likely to indicate or exacerbate depression, including personal or family history of depression, alcohol or drug use, stressful life events other than diagnosis of diabetes itself, and lack of social support, as well as previous episodes of depression and suicide attempts. Rule out organic causes of depression.

Since patients who express an initial depressive episode in response to the diagnosis of diabetes are at greater risk for a recurrence in the future, routine periodic screening for depression is recommended for these patients, especially if metabolic control deteriorates.

INSTITUTE EFFECTIVE TREATMENT FOR DEPRESSION AND ANXIETY DISORDER

Since depression and anxiety may be an acute response to metabolic disregulation and the emotional stress of diagnosis, supportive counseling by the clinician or psychotherapy by a qualified mental health professional are the initial treatments of choice. The choice of treatment or referral should be based upon the clinician's comfort in dealing with emotional problems and the apparent severity of the emotional distress.

If the emotional disorder does not resolve, consider the addition of psychotropic medication to the treatment regimen. Choosing the appropriate medication for patients with diabetes can be especially problematic because of potential side effects. For a discussion of available antidepressant medications and their side effects, see Chapter 15.

REFER TO MENTAL HEALTH PROFESSIONALS WHEN APPROPRIATE

Recognition of the importance of the emotional side of diabetes is growing. Especially with the increased demands of intensive treatment, emotional well-being is the foundation upon which all other aspects of the treatment regimen rest. The clinician can ensure that this emotional foundation is strong from the start by identifying and working with the problems and clinical syndromes discussed in this chapter and by recognizing the power of subclinical coping difficulties that are even more common among people with diabetes.

Sometimes, the clinician may feel that dealing with these issues is not possible because of limits in available time or skill. Under these circumstances, it is important to have a mental health referral source. Psychosocial treatment is a specialty in its own right. Try to identify a mental health specialist who has experience in treating people with diabetes. If such a person is not available, consider one who has experience treating patients with other chronic diseases or one who is interested in treating people with diabetes.

CONCLUSION

Effectively dealing with a newly diagnosed chronic disease, such as diabetes, requires a special kind of clinician-patient relationship. It is important for clinicians to help patients deal with emotional barriers to self-care from the time of diagnosis. These barriers, which range from denial, anger, and grief to obsessive-compulsive tendencies, anxiety, and depression, will be different for different individuals. Be sensitive to the existence of emotional responses to diagnosis and take active steps to help patients resolve any problematic responses.

BIBLIOGRAPHY

Hamburg BA, Inhoff GE: Coping with predictable crises of diabetes. *Diabetes Care* 6:409–416, 1983

Rubin RR, Biermann J, Toohey B: *Psyching out Diabetes.* Los Angeles, Lowell House, 1993

Rubin RR, Peyrot M: Psychosocial problems and interventions in diabetes. *Diabetes Care* 15:1640–1657, 1992

Using the Empowerment Approach to Help Patients Change Behavior

Robert M. Anderson, EdD, Martha M. Funnell, MS, RN, CDE, and Marilynn S. Arnold, MS, RD, CDE

INTRODUCTION

This chapter contains a method of helping patients change their behavior to improve their diabetes self-care and quality of life. The approach is based on sound principles of counseling and educational psychology, as well as the reality of the day-to-day management of a chronic disease such as diabetes. The empowerment approach requires a significant reexamination of the roles of health-care provider and patient. The new roles proposed herein are based on the significant differences between the treatment of acute disease and diabetes.

PRINCIPLES OF EMPOWERMENT

The empowerment approach is based on three key principles related to diabetes, its management, and the psychology of behavior change. The principles are summarized below.

1. The reality of diabetes care is that more than 98% of that care is provided by the patient; therefore, the patient is the locus of control and decision-making in the daily treatment of diabetes.
2. The primary mission of the health-care team is to provide ongoing diabetes expertise, education, and psychosocial support so

that patients can make informed decisions about their daily diabetes self-care.

3. Adults are much more likely to make and maintain behavior changes if those changes are personally meaningful and freely chosen.

ACUTE VS. CHRONIC DISEASE CARE

In the treatment of acute diseases, the health-care professional is the primary decision-maker and is generally in control of the treatment. The treatment of diabetes requires a different approach because it is a self-care disease. The health-care professional has two major responsibilities to the patient in the treatment of diabetes:

1. Provide the diabetes expertise required for the development of an effective diabetes self-care plan.
2. Provide the support and encouragement necessary for patients to make and sustain behavior changes designed to improve their diabetes care and quality of life.

These behavior changes need to be elicited from the patient rather than imposed by the health-care professional. This approach to diabetes care represents a significant change in the traditional relationship of patient and professional and requires new roles from both parties. Patients need to understand and ultimately accept that the daily care of their diabetes is their personal responsibility. Health-care professionals need to view their role as a consultant and the patient as the decision-maker.

HEALTH-CARE PROFESSIONAL BARRIERS TO USING EMPOWERMENT

There are two major barriers that many health-care professionals must overcome in order to successfully implement the empowerment approach to diabetes care.

1. The first barrier is the unwillingness or inability of some health-care professionals to elicit and explore the emotional content of a diabetes problem that a patient has identified. Having and car-

ing for diabetes has a potent emotional component for most patients. Adults seldom make and sustain significant changes in their lives unless they feel a strong need to change. If the change process is to be successful, it is crucial for the health professional to elicit the patient's feelings related to the potential behavior change. If the patient does not experience strong (usually negative) feelings about the current situation, the likelihood of sustained behavior change is small. Health-care professionals are not required to solve or change patients' emotions, but rather to create an environment in which the patient's emotional experience of the illness is validated and can be expressed freely.

2. The second major barrier is the tendency of many health-care professionals to solve problems for patients rather than with them. If a patient is clearly asking for technical expertise possessed by the health professional, such behavior is appropriate. For example, if a patient says "I don't know how to make my glucose meter work," the appropriate response is to teach the patient the required technique. However, most of the problems involved in the daily treatment of diabetes are more psychosocial than technical, e.g., "I find it really difficult to cut back on fat when my family insists on fried foods all the time." The solution to the second kind of problem must come from the patient if it is to be implemented successfully. The process of helping patients discover their capacity to solve their own problems reinforces their self-efficacy and personal responsibility for the treatment of their diabetes.

PATIENT BARRIERS TO USING EMPOWERMENT

There are major barriers that many patients must overcome in order to successfully implement this approach to diabetes care. Many patients are so used to being blamed and criticized for their efforts at diabetes self-care that they are reluctant to visit health-care professionals, discuss honestly their daily activities related to diabetes care, express any disagreement with a health-care professional, and assert their own needs or values related to the treatment of their diabetes. All of the above actions are necessary in order to develop and maintain an effective diabetes self-care plan. In order for health-care professionals to use the empowerment approach successfully, their patients need to believe that they are viewed as genuine partners in the care process.

PURPOSE

The following protocol is designed to help patients:

- Realize that they are responsible for and in charge of the daily treatment of their diabetes.
- Prioritize their diabetes-related problems and identify situations they want to improve.
- Experience the emotional and psychological commitment necessary to make and sustain a behavior change.
- Develop a behavior change plan.

BEHAVIOR CHANGE PROTOCOL

The following protocol is a series of questions to help patients identify and commit to a behavior change plan to improve their ability to live with and care for diabetes. The questions follow a logical sequence in terms of identifying problems and moving toward their solution. However, we are not suggesting that the questions be used as a rigid approach to interacting with patients. There are many situations in which the natural flow of the interaction would result in a discussion of the questions in a different order, the deletion of some questions, and/or the addition of other questions.

The questions below are meant to provide overall guidance in helping patients consider how they can improve their diabetes care. An important variable shaping the discussion will be how much the patient already knows about diabetes. There will be many instances when the health professional will need to provide information about diabetes care during the discussion. With some patients (especially newly diagnosed), the behavior change plan will focus on the acquisition of the information and skills necessary to make informed choices regarding diabetes care. These questions are meant to help support a process of patient-centered decision-making; however, we believe the clinician's judgment regarding the needs of the patient should be the major consideration guiding the interaction.

What part of living with diabetes is the most difficult or unsatisfying for you? (Would you tell me more about that? Would you give me some specific examples? Would you paint a picture of the situation for me?)

The purpose of this question is to focus the discussion on the patient's concerns about living with and caring for diabetes. Clinicians and patients often have different priorities about the most important issues related to diabetes care. Patients are most likely to change to solve problems that are personally meaningful and relevant to them.

How does that (the situation described above) make you feel? (Are you feeling [insert the feeling, e.g., angry, sad, confused, etc.]? Are you feeling [insert the feeling] because [insert the reason]?)

As mentioned earlier, patients seldom make and sustain changes in situations unless they care deeply about solving the problem or improving the situation. It is very common for people to repress uncomfortable emotions, and repressed emotions reduce the energy and clarity necessary for effective problem-solving.

Discussing the feelings associated with a particular diabetes care situation can energize patients. When patients experience the depth of their anger, sadness, or dissatisfaction by talking about their feelings, they are much more likely to take action in their own behalf.

How would this situation have to change for you to feel better about it? (Where would you like to be regarding this situation in [insert specific time, e.g., a month, 3 months]? What will happen if you don't do anything to change this situation? How will you feel if things don't change?)

The purpose of this question is to help patients identify concretely how the situation would appear if it were improved. This means imagining the particulars of the situation if it were to be changed and imagining how they would feel if the situation improved. It is also useful to help patients imagine how they would feel if things did not improve. This question helps patients focus on tangible elements in the situation that must change for them to feel better.

Are you willing to take action to improve the situation for yourself? (How important is it to you for this situation to improve?)

This question helps patients develop clarity about whether or not they are fully committed to changing the situation. It is a crucial question. However, in order for the question to have an impact, patients should feel free to make or not make a commitment to change. It is important that patients do not feel pressured to change to please the health-care professional, because changes made in response to such pressure seldom last.

What are some steps that you could take to bring you closer to where you want to be? (What could you do to help solve this problem? Are there any barriers you would have to overcome? Are there other people who could help you?)

This question helps patients develop a specific plan that will operationalize their commitment to change. It is useful to consider the various actions that could be taken, barriers to those actions, and potential resources, personal and otherwise, that patients could employ to help themselves.

Is there one thing that you will do when you leave here to improve things for yourself? This question brings the process to closure by focusing on the first thing the patient will do to begin to improve the situation. It is useful to come to closure by having identified at least one immediate step the patient will take to begin the problem-solving process. It is helpful, in many situations, to write down the action so that subsequent visits can include a discussion of how the problem-solving process proceeded and new strategies that can be made if the process was not successful. Patients may wish to take a written copy of a commitment to making a change with them when they leave the office. Commitments tend to be more binding when they are expressed publicly and documented.

If the answer to the last question is "Yes," I (the patient) will:

_____

_____

_____

_____

_____

_____

_____

CASE STUDIES

The following two case studies illustrate the traditional medical approach and the empowerment approach to helping patients change behavior. The case studies are condensed descriptions of patient-professional interactions. Actual transcripts of such transactions would be significantly longer. However, these condensed versions are meant to illustrate how the two approaches differ in the provision of diabetes care. The empowerment approach may require more time initially (as illustrated by the relative length of the two case studies) but is more likely to result in the identification of problems that are meaningful to the patient and strategies that are effective for long-term behavior change.

Case Study I: Traditional Medical Model Approach to Behavior Change

Patient: I hate this diet.

Professional: How many calories are you on?

Patient: 1,400. And I try so hard, but I just can't do it. My doctor bawls me out because I don't lose weight. I do pretty well at work all day, but then Joe comes home and wants a big dinner. And then we sit together and watch TV, and he wants me to bring him ice cream. And so I eat right along with him.

Professional: Why don't you try having your husband take a walk with you after dinner? And try eating yogurt instead of ice cream?

Patient: I tried yogurt before and I didn't like it very much. Also, I don't think Joe will be very interested in walking every night.

Professional: Try Fruity Delight Low-Fat Yogurt. It's great. And don't be so quick to give up on Joe walking. Will you at least give it a try?

Patient: Okay.

Professional: Great! I know you can do this if you really put your mind to it.

Case Study II: Empowerment Approach to Behavior Change

Patient: I hate this diet.

Professional: You sound pretty upset. Why don't you tell me about it.

Patient: I try so hard to cook like I am supposed to and eat what I was told. But, my husband refuses to eat that way and makes fun of me for being fat. Then, my doctor bawls me out for not losing weight. I have to give up what I like to eat, and then it still doesn't work.

Professional: That must be frustrating—to try so hard and not feel like you are getting anywhere.

Patient: It sure is. Why is it so hard to stick to this diet?

Professional: What do you think that the problem is?

Patient: Well, I do pretty well at work all day, but then Joe comes home and wants a big dinner. And then we sit together and watch TV, and he wants me to bring him ice cream. And so I eat right along with him.

Professional: What would have to change about this situation for you to feel better?

Patient: You know, I really do want to lose weight. Not just because my doctor told me, but because I don't like how I look and I don't have much energy to do the things I enjoy anymore.

Professional: What will happen if you don't change anything?

Patient: I'm not sure. I guess I'll gain more weight and my health will probably get worse, too.

Professional: How will you feel if that happens?

Patient: Awful. I'm just about at the end of my rope. I hate being frustrated and mad at myself all of the time. It's even affecting my work. And I'm crabby with the kids, too.

Professional: Can you accept things staying the way they are?

Patient: No! I've just got to lose some weight.

Professional: What is one thing you can do when you leave here to get you started?

Patient: I am going to talk to Joe. I can't believe he knows how bad I feel about the things he says. If I can just get him on my side, the battle would be half over.

Professional: When are you going to talk to him?

Patient: Tonight, when he gets home from work.

CONCLUSION

Change can be difficult for both health-care providers and patients. However, effective diabetes care requires new roles on the part of both parties. When appropriate changes in roles are made, both the health-care provider and the patient can find themselves part of a satisfying partnership that results in improved glycemic control for the patient and an enhanced sense of self-efficacy and level of satisfaction with care for both parties.

BIBLIOGRAPHY

Anderson RM: Patient empowerment and the traditional medical model: a case of irreconcilable differences? *Diabetes Care* 18:412–415, 1995

Anderson RM, Funnell MM, Butler P, Arnold MS, Fitzgerald JT, Feste C: Patient empowerment: results of a randomized control trial. *Diabetes Care* 18:943–949, 1995

Arnold MS, Butler PM, Anderson RM, Funnell MM, Feste C: Guidelines for facilitating a patient empowerment program. *The Diabetes Educator* 21:308–312, 1995

Feste C, Anderson RM: Empowerment: from philosophy to practice. *Patient Educ Counsel* 26:139–144, 1995

Funnell MM, Anderson RM, Arnold MS: Empowerment: a winning model for diabetes care. *Pract Diabetol* 10:15–18, 1991

Funnell MM, Anderson RM, Arnold MS, Barr PA, Donnelly MB, Johnson PD, Taylor-Moon D, White N: Empowerment: an idea whose time has come in diabetes education. *The Diabetes Educator* 17:37–41, 1991

Understanding and Treating Provider Burnout

18

Cindy L. Hanson, PhD

INTRODUCTION

Effective diabetes management requires considerable energy and endurance from providers as well as patients. Successful diabetes management involves individualized self-care goals, persistent problem-solving efforts based on the specific problems encountered by the patient, and ongoing provider support. These behaviors require time, persistence, enthusiastic endorsement, and flexibility in adapting to the individual needs of each patient. Despite concerted effort, treatment outcomes often fall short of the expectations of providers. Feelings of disappointment, frustration, and failure can lead to provider burnout. Patients can reciprocally reinforce these feelings of stress and defeat. Importantly, provider burnout disrupts an important therapeutic alliance for the patient. Several issues are discussed in this chapter:

- What is provider burnout?
- What are the signs of provider burnout?
- What causes burnout to develop?
- What can be done to prevent provider burnout?

WHAT IS PROVIDER BURNOUT?

Burnout is a psychological and physical response to chronic job stressors that occurs primarily in the caregiving, helping, or people-oriented professions. The chronic job stressors often involve 1) unrealistic job expectations and demands, and 2) nonreciprocated caregiving in emotionally draining and stressful situations. Definitions of burnout include negative changes in provider attitudes and behaviors as a result of chronic interpersonal and emotional stress at work. Sample definitions include:

- A state of physical, emotional, and mental exhaustion
- A progressive loss of idealism, energy, and purpose
- Feelings of helplessness and hopelessness, emotional drain, negative self-concept, and negative attitudes toward work, life, and other people
- Depleting one's physical and mental resources...by excessively striving to reach some unrealistic expectation imposed by oneself or by the values of society

Provider burnout generally results in a drain of provider energy and an inability to respond effectively to the demands of the job. Burnout is a process that develops over time and is best viewed on a continuum.

WHAT ARE THE SIGNS OF PROVIDER BURNOUT?

Provider burnout usually involves one or more of the following three characteristics:

1. Emotional exhaustion
2. Depersonalization
3. Reduced personal accomplishments

Emotional exhaustion refers to feelings of being emotionally overextended and depleted. Providers who work more hours and have overly excessive time demands are more likely to experience emotional exhaustion. Providers who are emotionally exhausted may try to reduce or minimize contact with patients. Many dysfunctional emotional patterns, such as frustration and irritation, can develop. Provider frustration and irritation with the patient can result in provider-patient distancing. Providers who are emotionally and physically drained are also less able to help change the patients' resources and environment in ways to facilitate the patients' control over their health and lives. Emotional and physical depletion can also create feelings of "compassion fatigue" in providers, which can result in detached responses to the needs, problems, and successes of patients.

Depersonalization is a term that is used to describe the impersonal and insensitive responses of providers who develop burnout. Providers can become callous and rude to staff and patients. Providers may also respond to patients with negative or fear messages because they may feel that it will help to motivate the patient. Any initial changes in behavior as a result of the negative messages are unlikely to be maintained in the long term, and they also become less effective in the short term. Negative messages also cause discomfort, hurt the provider-patient relationship, and contribute to provider burnout. They close people down rather than build them up.

Providers may depersonalize patients because of failures in treatment or because of a discomfort with the feelings and needs of patients. When providers become insensitive to the needs of patients, disengaged and ineffective therapeutic relationships develop. Providers may become disengaged and less sensitive to patients particularly when patients are experiencing failures and difficulties, which is unfortunately when the patients' needs are highest. This distance in the patient-provider relationship increases feelings of failure for both patients and providers. Patients need to feel accepted and supported, especially when they have failed to meet their own expectations and those of others. Failing within a supportive environment is an important part of the patients' acceptance of themselves and continued efforts toward self-management. If people feel supported and encouraged when they are unsuccessful with self-management techniques, they can more readily get back on track. By accepting the "lows" (within a context of encouraging the person's strengths and competencies and helping to facilitate a more supportive environment), people generally bounce back quicker and feel stronger than before. Provider burnout, however, inhibits this healing process.

Providers who feel professionally defeated are more likely to blame patients for poor health outcomes, which is another way of depersonalizing and distancing patients. Providers can hold misconceptions that place the blame (and subsequent guilt) for poor health on the individual patient. Providers may develop the attitude that patients do not want to get well or help themselves. Unless there are serious problems with low self-worth and depression, patients desire positive health and well-being and control over their lives. For patients who are experiencing low self-worth and depression, mental health providers can help strengthen this innate desire that may have been obstructed by physiological, personal, interpersonal, and/or contextual factors. Providers who have "tuned out" patients or are interacting with them in dysfunctional ways may not understand the patients' difficulties or detect the need for appropriate referrals.

Reduced personal accomplishment occurs when the provider withdraws and is unable to meet the demands of the job. A sense of incompetence, feelings of failure, and lack of job satisfaction can further escalate the burnout process. As a coping response, the provider may withdraw from job demands in order to maintain a sense of control and to preserve whatever resources and energy remain. Some providers do not experience a reduced sense of personal accomplishment in work as part of the burnout process, although they may experience a lowered sense of personal accomplishment and success in other family and social networks.

WHAT CAUSES PROVIDER BURNOUT TO DEVELOP?

Little, if any, research has been conducted on burnout among providers who care for people with diabetes. In searching the wider health-care literature, a few consistent patterns emerge as predictors of provider burnout. Provider burnout results from a combination of factors that interrelate with each other in complex ways:

- High job-related stresses (e.g., overcommitment, lack of staff support, inadequate funding and institutional support, low control over work demands, lack of job security)
- Low satisfaction in work and interpersonal relationships (e.g., dissatisfaction with workload, emotional exhaustion, poor relationships with colleagues and staff, low support from family and friends)
- Caregiving to patients with chronic or severe debilitating problems (e.g., cancer, AIDS, victims of abuse, chronic disease)

For providers who care for patients with diabetes, burnout is more likely to develop when:

- Unrealistic patient and provider goals and expectations have been set
- A consistent and positive approach toward the patient has not been used by the provider.
- Too much responsibility for the ongoing support and problem-solving has been undertaken by the provider rather than using the support systems in the patient's life and community
- Appropriate referrals and resources have been underutilized

WHAT CAN BE DONE TO PREVENT PROVIDER BURNOUT?

There are several prevention strategies that might be useful for provider burnout:

Be sensitive to feelings, beliefs, attitudes, and biases; and be open to appropriate feedback from caring family and friends. With provider burnout, the provider not only becomes less sensitive to the patient but also becomes less aware of his or her own feelings of disengagement that are undermining the provider's treatment efforts with patients. Colleagues often experience similar stressful work demands, and they may share "blind spots" regarding the emotional and physical costs of chronic work stress. Family members and friends can help the provider recognize the effects of the escalating stress. The provider can then identify those areas that are contributing to the problem and can seek solutions.

Set realistic goals that allow for normal fluctuations in disease management throughout the course of the patient's life. Both patients and providers need to recognize the small successes and be prepared for the chronicity of the disease and the demands that are placed on them. Provider characteristics, such as "noble aspirations" and "high initial provider enthusiasm," have predicted provider burnout, likely because expectations were set too high relative to the resources available and the nature of the disease. Providers who ask patients what goals they wish to achieve and help devise specific plans to obtain only one or two of these goals at a time are more likely to experience success versus burnout.

Understand developmental life stages and demands in order to develop appropriate expectations, recognize sources of stress, and provide anticipatory guidance to patients. Patients vacillate between stages in dealing with their disease, largely because of developmental and life milestones. If the provider understands the developmental challenges that patients face, he or she will be better able to set realistic expectations, provide appropriate anticipatory guidance to patients, and help avoid burnout. From a developmental perspective, it is also important for the provider to recognize that he or she may experience a reevaluation of life goals and career choice in midlife, or after 10 to 15 years in practice. During this readjustment period, problems associated with burnout, occupational stress, and job dissatisfaction may be intensified.

Operate under the premise that the primary task is not to be the sole provider, but rather to help the patient develop a professional and personal support network to help with the individualized diabetes-related goals (see below).

Incorporate family and other support systems as an essential part of the treatment plan and goals. Providers may not engage the family or other support networks in the treatment plan because their goal is for patients to feel more internally motivated. Self-motivation, however, develops primarily through encouragement by others and a positive sense of self and competency. Providers can help patients with self-motivation through a focus on the strengths of the person and by providing guidance and referrals needed for supportive resources (e.g., financial, family, recreational, and community). Family members and friends need to understand what types of support the person desires, when support is needed (e.g., at home, at work, around friends, in public places), and how often the person desires the supportive behaviors (see Chapter 19).

Identify referral sources and develop a team approach to care. A consistent factor that emerges in the literature to help prevent provider burnout is having collaborative support from other health professionals. If a team approach is unavailable, the provider can consult with other health professionals to build a network of referral sources. Support from even a few colleagues can help. Sharing provider-patient experiences and problems with other providers can help to alleviate the stress that leads to burnout, and it often provides new insights on ways to solve ongoing problems. One way that colleagues can help is by identifying difficulties in the patients' lives to which the provider may have become insensitive. The colleagues' previous experiences with similar problems may be helpful.

Use resources for diabetes-related and lifestyle support. There are many community and national resources for diabetes information:

- American Diabetes Association (ADA: 1-800-342-2383)
- Juvenile Diabetes Foundation (JDF: 1-800-223-1138)
- National Diabetes Information Clearinghouse (NDIC: 1-301-654-3327 for patients; 1-800-891-5388 for providers)
- American Association for Diabetes Educators (AADE: 1-800-TEAM-UP #4 [832-6874] for patients; 1-800-338-3633 for providers)

Providers and patients can call the ADA and the JDF to gain information about local or regional chapters of the organizations and to obtain booklets and brochures about diabetes and its management, as well as late-breaking news. Membership benefits for providers and patients include subscriptions to patient-oriented books and magazines (*Diabetes Forecast* from the ADA and *Countdown* from the JDF), as well as professional books and journals for providers. Local or regional ADA chapters can provide information about diabetes camps, support groups, and educational seminars in the area. The NDIC disseminates booklets and pamphlets about all aspects of diabetes for both patients and providers. Providers can call the AADE for local chapter news, newsletters, conferences, and educational seminars. Patients can call the AADE to receive names of local diabetes educators in their areas.

Other resources include an excellent monthly newspaper for providers and patients called the *Diabetes Interview* (3715 Balboa Street, San Francisco, CA 94121; 415-387-4002). Local libraries, hospitals, or newspapers have information on community resources, such as family workshops, exercise and weight-management programs, informational health fairs, and support groups for people with diabetes. Pharmaceutical companies have patient brochures related to diabetes education and management. Many of the major pharmaceutical companies will also financially support educational seminars and groups.

Strive for balance. In order to avoid burnout, providers who have heavy and demanding schedules need to care for their own physical and emotional health, and they need to pace themselves so that their work is balanced with other sources of support and pleasure.

CONCLUSION

As suggested throughout this chapter, health-care providers are only one component of successful disease management. It is essential that health-care providers not only engage in one-on-one teaching, helping, encouraging, and strengthening, but also use their expertise to facilitate these types of interpersonal relationships in the patient's life to avoid burnout. Successful diabetes management requires the support and integration of the key people in the patient's life, as well as more wide-scale community and national efforts to reduce the financial and emotional burdens of care on the patients and providers.

BIBLIOGRAPHY

Glasgow RE: A practical model of diabetes management and education. *Diabetes Care* 18:117–126, 1995

Hanson CL: The health of children with IDDM: a shift to family-centered, community-based care. *Diabetes Spectrum* 7:390–392, 1994

Maslach C: Stress, burnout, and workaholism. In *Professionals in Distress: Issues, Syndromes, and Solutions in Psychology.* Kilburg RR, Nathan PE, Thoreson RW, Eds. Washington, DC, American Psychological Association, 1986, p. 53–75

McKegney CP: Surviving survivors: coping with caring for patients who have been victimized. *Primary Care* 20:481–494, 1993

Papatheodorou NH (Ed.): Interactive communication in health-care delivery. *Diabetes Spectrum* 3:217–256, 1990

Sauter SL, Murphy LR, Hurrell JJ: Prevention of work-related psychological disorders: a national strategy proposed by the National Institute for Occupational Safety and Health (NIOSH). *Am Psychol* 45:1146–1158, 1990

Sims DF, Sims AH (Eds.): Motivation, adherence, and the therapeutic alliance. *Diabetes Spectrum* 2:17–52, 1989

Snibbe JR, Radcliffe T, Weisberger C, Richards M, Kelly J: Burnout among primary care physicians and mental health professionals in a managed health care setting. *Psychol Rep* 65:775–780, 1989

Understanding and Treating Patients With Diabetes Burnout

19

William H. Polonsky, PhD, CDE

INTRODUCTION

Mrs. J is a 54-year-old secretary with a 6-year history of type II diabetes. Frightened by the possibility of long-term complications, she has always been anxious about managing her diabetes. She was relatively successful in the first months following diagnosis, but she became increasingly frustrated with her prescribed meal plan, which she found quite restrictive, and with her inability to establish a regular schedule for daily walking. Despite her best efforts, she was unable to lose weight as directed (partly because of her new oral hypoglycemic agent) and experienced several frightening episodes of mild hypoglycemia. Over the years, her attempts at self-management have slowly deteriorated. At this time, she continues to take her oral medication faithfully each day, but she tests her blood glucose only rarely (approximately only once a week). As she notes, "Why bother testing at all? It's always too high!" She continues to follow her prescribed meal plan, at least through the early parts of the day. By suppertime, however, she begins to binge, which continues unchecked until bedtime. Regular physical activity is no longer even attempted. Her husband and close friends are constantly pushing her to "try harder," but this has not been helpful and has only increased her sense of isolation with diabetes. She tries not to think about her illness and avoids seeing her physician, who she fears will recommend that she begin insulin. When she does think about diabetes, she feels angry and frustrated with herself, feeling overwhelmed, exhausted, and defeated by her diabetes and very worried about her future health. Mrs. J is suffering with diabetes burnout.

WHAT IS DIABETES BURNOUT?

Burnout was originally conceptualized as a common response to a chronically difficult and frustrating job, where the individual works harder and harder each day and yet has little sense that these actions are making a real difference. The individual may feel chronically overextended and depleted, and there may be a sense of inadequacy or guilt that he or she is failing at the job. Feelings of helplessness, hopelessness, irritability, and hostility are also common, resulting in a state of chronic emotional exhaustion.

As in Mrs. J's case, the experience of living with diabetes may commonly lead to feelings of burnout. The patient may come to feel that the day-to-day vigilance and effort expended to properly manage diabetes is too burdensome and frustrating and the results too inconsequential to make the effort worthwhile. Feeling overwhelmed and defeated by diabetes, the patient may still worry that he or she is not taking care of diabetes well enough and yet feel unable, unmotivated, or unwilling to change. At its roots, diabetes burnout is about hopelessness and poor self-efficacy, i.e., the patient's sense that he or she cannot achieve and/or maintain appropriate diabetes self-care, even while believing it to be an important goal.

WHY WORRY ABOUT DIABETES BURNOUT?

While the prevalence of diabetes burnout is not yet known, we suspect that it may be relatively common. In two recent studies, we found that diabetes-specific emotional distress was widespread among clinic patients at a large diabetes center, with approximately 60% of the patients sampled reporting at least one serious diabetes-related concern.

Those patients who report higher levels of diabetes burnout (chronic frustration and feelings of failure) tend to have significantly higher glycosylated hemoglobin levels and to report significantly poorer self-care.

Diabetes burnout may be much more prevalent in patients who have dropped out of medical care. By definition, patients with diabetes burnout have compromised their diabetes self-care such that chronically elevated blood glucose levels are common and, consequently, long-term complications are more likely to occur. Tragically, many of these patients may be seen only rarely by health-care providers until complications begin to emerge. We suspect that future research will document that diabetes burnout is a major risk factor for poor glycemic control and the consequent, perhaps early, onset of long-term diabetes complications. If diabetes burnout can be identified, understood, and treated in clinic populations and, hopefully, in harder-to-reach populations, we believe that this could potentially contribute to improving long-term glycemic control and reducing rates of long-term complications in a substantial subgroup of patients.

SIX STRATEGIES FOR ALLEVIATING DIABETES BURNOUT

To alleviate diabetes burnout and assist patients in maintaining better self-care, six major strategies are recommended. These strategies are somewhat overlapping and may be considered to be additive in their efficacy.

Learn to Recognize Diabetes Burnout

Assessment of diabetes burnout can be difficult, since patients may be unable to easily recognize their own complex feelings about diabetes, or they may feel embarrassed to discuss their feelings with health-care providers, whom they may perceive (rightly or wrongly) as judgmental. Make it comfortable for patients to be honest about the aggravation and distress that often accompany diabetes self-care by normalizing it. For example, rather than asking, "You're not having any problems with managing your diabetes, are you?," consider saying, "Everyone struggles with managing their diabetes from time to time, what's that struggle like for you?" A patient with diabetes burnout may have any of the following signs or symptoms:

- Patient feels that diabetes is controlling (or trying to control) his or her life.
- Patient feels overwhelmed by self-care goals and actions, and usually feels that he or she is failing with diabetes.
- Patient has strong, negative feelings about diabetes.
- Patient feels alone with diabetes, that no one understands.
- Patient admits to chronically poor self-care and poor glycemic control (brief episodes of excellent control may also occur).
- Patient has seen health-care providers very infrequently; may have no record of regular, ongoing care.
- Patient reports strong ambivalence about improving self-care (may feel that proper self-management is not worth the effort, but feels guilty and/or frightened about his or her history of poor self-care).

Establish a Strong, Collaborative Relationship With Patients

Patients with diabetes burnout often anticipate an adversarial relationship with their health-care provider, feeling certain that they will be judged, demeaned, and/or treated disrespectfully. Thus, they may be somewhat withdrawn or avoidant during sessions, and they may tend to postpone, cancel, or altogether avoid appointments with health-care providers. Such feelings and expectations may not be totally unreasonable, given that these patients may have had previous negative interactions with significant others (including health-care providers) about their diabetes. To intervene effectively, it is essential to be respectful of the patient's struggle with diabetes self-care. Clearly delineate the areas of responsibility for the patient, clarifying that the provider can serve as an advisor only and strongly encouraging active patient participation in all decision-making, goal-setting, and problem-solving. It is important to avoid an overly authoritarian or parental attitude (see Chapter 17 on empowerment). Focus on promoting adherence (referring to the patient's interest in reaching a desired treatment goal) rather than compliance (referring to the patient's obedience to the provider's instructions). To encourage a collaborative relationship, even office geography may play a role. For example, sitting next to the patient, rather than behind a desk, may help to promote a less authoritarian relationship.

In a meeting with a diabetes burnout patient, take time to review all self-care behaviors. As goals are established (see below), remember to help the patient identify where he or she is successful, not just where self-care shortcomings may lie. Also, pay respectful attention to the patient's blood glucose records. No matter how meager such records may be, if the patient is able to prepare and share records, consider the records and discuss them with the patient. Indeed, giving thoughtful attention to records is such a considerate and respectful gesture toward all patients that it may be one of the best predictors of whether the patient continues to bring records to future sessions.

Since alleviating diabetes burnout is likely to take time, a supportive and concerned provider will be most effective when continuity of regular care and contact is established. As described earlier, the patient with diabetes burnout may tend to avoid or cancel appointments, especially when he or she is discouraged with self-care (e.g., "I've kept so few records that there's no need to go to my appointment; my doctor will just be angry with me anyway."). Thus, when the patient and provider can proactively schedule a series of regular visits over 6 to 12 months and there is a clearly stated agreement that the patient will attend these visits, regardless of his or her "success" at self-care, the patient is more likely to feel respected and cared about, that self-care is important, and that he or she is an important (and responsible) member of the health-care team.

At first, the less time between scheduled visits, the better. And, when at all possible, follow-up contacts between visits (e.g., phone calls, faxing of patient blood glucose records, provider letters and reinforcing comments to the patient) are very valuable. One patient, for example, stated that the most important factor in ending her years of diabetes burnout was one particular action of her new physician. Between her first and second visit, he phoned her several times (once a week) to check on her progress. By this unique action alone, she began to feel cared about and respected, and, subsequently, she began to care more about herself and her diabetes.

Negotiate Goals

When self-care goals are unclear and/or unreasonable, diabetes burnout is more likely to occur. Help patients identify their current expectations and assist them in developing new self-care goals that are more concrete and more achievable. Mrs. J, for example, had been told that walking each day was absolutely essential for her diabetes management. While she had no clear sense of how many miles were necessary to be successful, she did feel that she was "failing" every day (she was averaging 1 mile, 4 days a week). After further discussion, she realized that she had somehow decided that the minimum for "successful" walking was 3 miles, 7 days a week. To prevent her from giving up her walking program completely (which she was close to doing), the provider assisted her in selecting a target for weekly walking that was more reasonable for her (1 mile, 5 days a week), a goal that helped her to feel successful and upon which she could gradually build more challenging goals. To promote "success experiences," diabetes self-care goals must be concrete, specific, time-limited, uncomplicated, measurable, and—most importantly—realistic.

Pay Attention to Strong, Negative Feelings About Diabetes

In diabetes burnout, goal planning and other behavioral interventions are not likely to be successfully implemented when the patient is so guilt-ridden, despondent, angry, or fearful about diabetes that he or she does not feel hopeful that such actions will be valuable. Take time to hear and acknowledge the patient's difficult feelings about diabetes. Toward this end, it is essential to put aside preconceived notions about how the patient may feel and make sure to ask directly about diabetes-related distress (e.g., "How is diabetes driving you crazy?") and to ascertain how the patient makes sense of diabetes (e.g., "How do you feel about having diabetes?," "Do you think taking care of your diabetes is worth doing?," "Are you worried about the possibility of complications?"). And listening well and respectfully, rather than leaping quickly to find solutions for the patient's feelings, may be the most important step. The provider's most important response should be to normalize the patient's negative feelings about diabetes, reassuring the patient that such feelings are common and understandable.

Optimize Social Support

The patient with diabetes burnout may feel quite isolated with diabetes, believing that no one understands or appreciates the struggle with the illness. When the patient begins to feel supported, that a friend, family member, or health-care provider is truly understanding and actively rooting for him or her, diabetes burnout may begin to dissipate. To promote more valuable support, there are three major problem-solving interventions to employ: 1) add positive support behaviors, 2) eliminate negative support behaviors, and 3) clarify regimen responsibilities.

First, ask the patient to consider the idiosyncratic ways, no matter how silly, selfish, or unrealistic these may at first seem, in which family and friends might be of more direct assistance in managing diabetes. This includes emotional as well as behavioral support.

While the patient may benefit by thinking of creative ways in which to ask friends and family to help, he or she may also profit by considering those ongoing behaviors of significant others that are not helpful and need to be stopped. Diabetes burnout may be more likely when the patient's spouse downplays the difficulty and importance of diabetes care; demanding, for example, that cookies and candy be available in the house for all other family members and telling the patient to "just use willpower" to avoid these sweets. Also, friends, family, and health-care providers may serve as "diabetes police," choosing to "help" the patient manage diabetes, regardless of whether the patient may want such assistance! When the patient feels hounded by such infantilizing comments as "You shouldn't be eating that," "You seem upset, maybe you should check your blood sugars," or "If you want to lose weight, you better start applying more self-discipline," the patient may begin to withdraw from significant others, becoming more isolated and discouraged. By encouraging the patient to confront significant others, in as creative and tactful a manner as possible, and find ways to redirect their "helpfulness" into more beneficial actions (see Chapter 5 on involving families), self-care may improve and diabetes burnout may be significantly reduced. For example, Mrs. J asked her husband to stop constantly recommending that she "try harder" and, instead, requested that he join her in regular evening activities (e.g., a walk through the neighborhood) that might distract her from binge eating.

Finally, consider the potential value of a family meeting, especially when there is apparent confusion about who is responsible for each self-care activity.

Engage Patients in Active Problem-Solving

When considering an intervention for a patient with diabetes burnout, consider these four major aspects of problem-solving.

First, since feeling overwhelmed is a central facet of diabetes burnout, limit any planned change in the self-care regimen to one self-care behavior at a time (following from the discussion above, this increases the likelihood of a "success experience"). For example, Mr. F, a 39-year-old man with type I diabetes, decided that, after years of diabetes burnout and very poor self-care, he was ready to begin managing his diabetes "perfectly." Rather than support such a large and rapid change of behavior, the patient was encouraged to start with only one selected change before moving on to his other goals.

Second, make the initial focus of any planned change in self-care, especially if it involves a behavior that has not been a routine part of the patient's lifestyle in some time, on building that behavior into a regularly established habit. For Mr. F, who chose to begin with regular blood glucose testing, this was certain to be an important area of concern, because over the past 5 years he had tested his blood glucose levels on a very irregular basis (approximately once a month). Thus, the focus of the initial intervention was solving how he could begin testing regularly prebreakfast, including how he would remember to do so (e.g., what other morning event he could link his testing to) as well as how he would make sure to have the time available each morning (e.g., setting his alarm to arise 10 minutes earlier each morning).

Third, as possible solutions to a problem are considered, keep in mind the patient's previous successes with a similar problem. For example, in the previous year, Mr. F had succeeded in restructuring his morning ritual so that he would remember to take his vitamins at breakfast (he placed the vitamins next to the coffeepot). He adapted this solution to successfully establish the habit of A.M. blood glucose testing (he placed his meter next to his shaving kit).

Fourth, consider simple environmental solutions first. These tend to be the easiest to adopt. Mr. F could have been encouraged to use his "willpower" to remember his testing each morning, but he was more likely to be successful if he followed the clinician's suggestions for simple concrete adjustments in his environment (e.g., leave your meter next to your shaving kit, set your alarm 10 minutes earlier).

CONCLUSION

In conclusion, diabetes can be a difficult and burdensome illness, and feelings of distress are common. When the negative consequences of diabetes self-care are perceived as too burdensome, diabetes burnout may result. Diabetes burnout is characterized by feelings of being overwhelmed and defeated by diabetes, a sense of hopelessness that appropriate diabetes self-care cannot be achieved and/or maintained, and— consequently—poor self-care and chronically elevated blood glucose levels. We suspect that a substantial subgroup of patients may be suffering (albeit silently) with diabetes burnout. Therefore, proper identification and treatment of diabetes burnout may be very important. Six major strategies for treating diabetes burnout were presented. It is hoped that future research will point to a more refined description of diabetes burnout, better evidence as to the actual prevalence and consequences of diabetes burnout, and a more comprehensive (and experimentally rigorous) set of treatment strategies.

BIBLIOGRAPHY

Cox DJ, Gonder-Frederick LA: Major developments in behavioral diabetes research. *J Consult Clin Psychol* 60:628–638, 1992

Goodall TA, Halford WK: Self-management of diabetes mellitus: a critical review. *Health Psychol* 10:1–8, 1991

Greenfield S, Kaplan SH, Ware JE, Yano EM, Frank HJL: Patients' participation in medical care: effects on blood sugar control and quality of life in diabetes. *J Gen Intern Med* 3:448–457, 1988

Hoover JW: Patient 'burnout' can explain non-compliance. In *World Book of Diabetes in Practice*. Vol. 3. Krall LP, Ed. New York, Elsevier Science Publishers, 1988

Kurtz SMS: Adherence to diabetes regimens: empirical status and clinical applications. *The Diabetes Educator* 16:50–56, 1990

Meichenbaum D, Turk D: *Facilitating Treatment Adherence.* New York, Plenum, 1987

Polonsky WH: Psychosocial aspects of diabetes. In *Psychophysiological Disorders.* Gatchel R, Blanchard E, Eds. Washington, DC, American Psychological Association, 1993

Polonsky WH, Anderson BJ, Lohrer PA, Welch G, Jacobson AM, Schwartz C: Assessment of diabetes-specific distress. *Diabetes Care* 18:754–760, 1995

Polonsky WH, Welch GM: Listening to our patients' concerns: understanding and addressing diabetes-specific emotional distress. *Diabetes Spectrum* 9:8–11, 1996

Rubin RR, Biermann J, Toohey B: *Psyching Out Diabetes.* Los Angeles, Lowell House, 1992

Welch G, Jacobson AM, Polonsky WH: Attitudinal predictors of the emotional impact of diabetes mellitus. *Diabetes* 44 (Suppl. 1):259A, 1995

AFTERWORD

In closing, we would like to note several of the important themes that appear throughout the pages of this book.

First, patients and their families assume most of the responsibility for following and adjusting the diabetes regimen, and these responsibilities are carried out within a complicated emotional, behavioral, and social context that is unique to each individual.

Second, all members of the health-care team are responsible for the psychological support of patients with diabetes and their families, and all clinical interactions affect patients' psychological well-being.

Third, clinicians are encouraged to take a balanced, realistic approach to diabetes self-care, avoiding interventions that may be experienced by patients as judgmental. Patients who develop the capacity for flexible problem-solving, accepting occasional lapses in management as a fact of life, often find the disease less oppressive and maintain improved metabolic control.

Fourth, knowledge of diabetes and its treatment does not ensure adherence to a self-care regimen, and adherence, in turn, does not ensure normoglycemia.

Finally, in many instances, the services of a mental health professional who has knowledge of diabetes and its treatment can be invaluable.

We hope that this book meets the goal we set in creating it: to make the latest psychological knowledge related to diabetes attainable and applicable.

Barbara J. Anderson, PhD
Richard R. Rubin, PhD, CDE

INDEX

A

Activity levels. *See also* Exercise
 glycemic control and, 5–6, 66–67
 profile of, 78, 80
Adherence problems, in adolescents,
 31–32
Adolescents, 13–33
 adherence problems, 31–32
 contact, maintaining, 19–20
 DCCT results for, 15, 23–24
 developmental considerations, 24,
 137–138
 eating disorders and. *See* Eating disorders
 emotional strength, building, 20–21
 endocrinologic effects of puberty, 25
 exercise and, 27–28
 feelings, dealing with, 16–17,
 136–138
 glycemic control, 15, 17–19
 intensive, 23–24, 30–33
 hypoglycemia and, 30
 insulin regimens for, 25–26
 insulin resistance, 25
 mental health service referrals,
 21–22
 metabolic reactivity, 138–139
 nutrition, 26–27
 peer support groups, 137–138
 problem-solving skills, 20, 26
 self-care readiness, 13–14, 30–32

self-monitoring of blood glucose
 (SMBG), 28–29
 specificity, need for, 18–19
 treatment goals, 17–19, 29
Aging. *See* Elderly patients
Alcohol, hypoglycemic symptoms and,
 86–87
Anger, 157, 188
Anorexia nervosa, 133
Antidepressants, 149–151
Anxiety disorder, 159–161
Autonomic neuropathy, exercise
 risks/recommendations, 79
Autonomic symptoms, of hypo-
 glycemia, 86–87, 90, 94

B

Beck Depression Inventory (BDI), 148
Behavior management techniques
 in children, 7–9
 empowerment. *See* Empowerment
 for weight control, 118
Beliefs, of patients, self-management
 and, 56–57
Blame
 by family members, 45
 by providers, 175–176
Blood glucose awareness training
 (BGAT), 52, 83, 91
Bulimia nervosa, 133

Burnout
  patient, 183–192
    defined, 184
    negative feelings and, 188
    prevalence, 184–185
    problem-solving aspects, 190
    recognizing, 185–186
    relationship with provider,
      186–187
    self-care goals, 187–188
    social support, 188–189
    symptoms, 186
    treatment, 185–190
  provider, 173–181
    causes, 176–177
    compassion fatigue, 175
    defined, 174
    depersonalization, 175–176
    emotional exhaustion, 174–175
    prevention, 177–180
    reduced personal accomplish-
      ment, 176
    signs of, 174–176

C

Carbohydrates, low blood glucose and,
  95–96
Catastrophizing, 157
Children, 3–11
  diagnosis, critical issues at, 3–4
  glycemic control in, 5–6
  hypoglycemia in, 5–6
  parental intervention, 6–9
  self-esteem of, 6
  self-management and, 4, 7–9
  social adjustment of, 6
  treatment guidelines, 3–6
Chronic disease care, 164
Clinicians. See Health-care team
Cognitive therapy (CT), for depression, 151
Compassion fatigue, 175
Complications. See also Heart
    disease; Nephropathy;
    Neuropathy; Retinopathy
  in adolescents, reducing, 29
  depression and, 144–146
  diabetes burnout and, 185
  exercise risks/recommendations,
    79

fears about, 46–47
  smoking and, 121
Computerized assessment, of self-
    management issues, 58–61
Costs
  family concerns about, 45
  of intensive therapy, 31
Counseling
  for eating disorder prevention,
    135–140
  nutritional, 27
  for smoking cessation, 124,
    125–126
Counterregulation, decreased, 86–87

D

Denial, 156–157
Depersonalization, provider, 175–176
Depression, 143–152
  antidepressants, 149–151
  Beck Depression Inventory (BDI),
    148
  causes of, 144
  complications and, 144–146
  diagnosis of, 146–148
  at diagnosis of diabetes, 159–161
  in elderly patients, 40–41
  electroconvulsive therapy and, 151
  hyperglycemia and, 159
  hypoglycemia and, 146
  interaction with diabetes, 144–146,
    159–160
  prevalence, 143–144
  screening for, 159–161
  subclinical, 157
  treatment, 148–151
Diabetes burnout. See Burnout, patient
Diabetes Control and Complications
    Trial (DCCT), 6, 27, 105
  glycated hemoglobin levels, in ado-
    lescents, 15, 23–24
  glycemic control for adolescents,
    23–24
  hypoglycemia and, 30, 52
Diabetes Quality of Life (DQOL), 107
Diabetic ketoacidosis (DKA), eating
    disorders and, 135
Diagnosis, of diabetes
  critical issues at, 3–4, 155
Diary, blood glucose, 98, 100–101

Dietary self-management. *See* Nutritional management

E

Ease of access index, for exercise, 77
Ease of performance index, for exercise, 77–78
Eating disorders, 133–141
  anorexia nervosa, 133
  bulimia nervosa, 133
  family involvement, 139
  forms of, 133
  metabolic reactivity, 138–139
  negative feelings and, 136–138
  prevalence, 134
  prevention, 135–140
  stress and, 135
  warning signs, 134–135
Eating habits. *See* Nutritional management
Education, diabetes, 6–7
  for family members, 44, 47–49
  for intensive therapy, 106
  nutritional counseling, 27
  resources, 179–180
  self-management training, 7–9, 26
Elderly patients, 35–42
  aging
    developmental tasks of, 35–36
    perspective on, 37
  clinician's attitudes towards, 36
  depression in, 40–41
  family support for, 40
  functional status of, 37–38
  goal-setting, 39–40
  self-care, barriers to, 38–39
Emotional exhaustion, provider, 174–175
Emotional strength, in adolescents, 20–21
Emotions. *See also* Burnout; Depression
  adolescents and, 16–17
  anger, 157, 188
  eating disorders and, 136–138
  of family members, 45–47
  fear. *See* Fears
  mood changes, with hypoglycemia, 88–89, 90
  problems at diagnosis, 157–158

sadness (subclinical depression), 157
smoking cessation and, 127–130
stress. *See* Stress
Empowerment, 163–172
  barriers to
    health-care team, 164–165
    patient, 165–166
  case studies, 169–171
  eating disorders and, 139–140
  principles of, 163–164
  protocol for, 166–168
  vs. traditional approach, 169–171
Epinephrine secretion, 86, 89
Exercise
  activity profile, 78, 80
  adolescents and, 27–28
  benefits, 27, 74, 75
  complications and, 78–79
  ease of access index, 77
  ease of performance index, 77–78
  goal-setting, 81
  hypoglycemia and, 27–28, 80, 95, 96
  motivating factors, 74–76, 78, 80–81
  program selection, 76–77
  reinforcement, 74–75
  unplanned, 28
  weight control and, 114–115
Expectations
  of family members, 47–48
  of patient-centered management, 67–68

F

Family members, 43–50
  adolescents and, 15, 31
  diabetes burnout and, 188–189
  eating disorders and, 135, 139
  emotional problems at diagnosis and, 158
Fears
  diabetes burnout and, 188
  of family members, 46–47, 85
  of hypoglycemia, 85–86
  responses to
    catastrophizing, 157
    denial, 156–157
Financial concerns
  of family members, 45
  intensive therapy costs, 31

Functional status, of elderly patients, 37–38

G

Glucose tablets or gel, 99–100
Glycated hemoglobin (HbA$_1$ or HbA$_{1c}$)
    elevated, 135
    intensive therapy and, 15, 23–24
    nephropathy risk and, 29
Glycemic control. *See also*
        Hypoglycemia
    in adolescents, 15, 17–19, 23–33
    blood glucose awareness training
        (BGAT), 52, 83, 91
    in children, 5–6
    depression and, 144–146
    family member expectations, 47–48
    goals, biochemical, 29
    improving, 23–33, 105–111
        empowerment approach, 166–171
    intensive therapy
        for adolescents, 23–24, 30–33
        changing to, 106–107
        health–care team, demands on,
            107, 109–110
        hypoglycemia and, 30
        obsessive–compulsive tendencies,
            158–159
        psychological factors, 108–109
        trial period, 108
    weight loss and, 114
Guilt, of family members, 45

H

Health-care team
    acute *vs.* chronic disease care, 164
    burnout. *See* Burnout, provider
    elderly patients, attitudes toward, 36
    empowerment, barriers to, 164–165
    intensive therapy, demands of, 107,
        109–110
    patient-centered care and, 70–71
    relationships with patients, 186–187
        adolescents, 16–18
    responsibilities of, 164
    self-management assessment,
        55–61
    smoking cessation, 122–123,
        130–131
Health insurance, 45

Heart disease
    depression and, 144
    nutritional management and, 69
    smoking and, 121
Honeymoon phenomenon, 7, 26
Humor, 21
Hyperglycemia
    in children, 5–6
    depression and, 146, 159
Hypnosis, for smoking cessation, 127
Hypoglycemia, 83–102. *See also* Low
        blood glucose
    in adolescents, 30
    blood glucose awareness training
        (BGAT), 52, 83, 91
    in children, 5–6
    exercise and, 27–28, 80, 95–96
    fear of, 46–47, 85–86
    intensive therapy and, 30
    mild, 83–85
    mood changes, 88–89, 90
    prevention, 94–97
    severe, 83–85, 93–102
        eating disorders and, 135
        low blood glucose events and,
            93–94
    symptoms, 85–91
        alcohol and, 86–87
        autonomic, 86–87, 90, 94
        depression and, 146
        neuroglycopenic, 87–90
        recognizing, 89–91
    unawareness of, 91

I

Independent diabetes care. *See* Self-
        management
Insulin omission, eating disorders and,
        135
Insulin regimens
    adjustment of, 66–67
    for adolescents, 25–26
    exercise and, 28
    hypoglycemia prevention and, 94–95
Insulin resistance, in adolescents, 25
Intensive therapy. *See* Glycemic
        control
Interpersonal therapy (IPT), for
        depression, 151